PE·METRICS™

Assessing
National Standards 1-6
In Secondary School

Published by

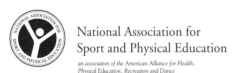

National Association for
Sport and Physical Education
an association of the American Alliance for Health,
Physical Education, Recreation and Dance

NASPE Sets the Standard

1900 Association Drive, Reston, Va. 20191 (703) 476-3410 www.naspeinfo.org

To order more copies of this book (stock # 304-10504):

Web: www.naspeinfo.org
E-mail: customerservice@aahperd.org
Phone: (800) 321-0789; (412) 741-1288 outside the United States
Fax: (412) 741-0609
Mail: AAHPERD Publications Fulfillment Center, P.O. Box 1020, Sewickley, PA 15143-1020

ISBN: 978-0-88314-960-7

Printed in the United States

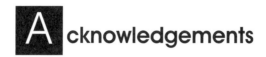 # Acknowledgements

Assessment Task Force

Marybell Avery
Ben Dyson
Jennifer L. Fisette
Connie Fox
Marian Franck
Kim C. Graber
Judith H. Placek, chair
Judith Rink
Lori Williams
Weimo Zhu

Technical Assistance

Marco Boscolo
Connie Fox
Pamela MacFarlane
Sara Khosravi Nasr
Youngsik Park
Eng Wah Teo
Weimo Zhu

NASPE Staff

Charlene Burgeson, Executive Director
Cheryl Richardson, Senior Program Manager
Joe McGavin, Publications Manager

NASPE extends its appreciation to the many professionals who served as project administrators and coders in the gathering of thousands of pieces of individual student data for the secondary-level Standard 1 assessments. That list includes: Ann Arns, Marybell Avery, Deb Berkey, Tim Bott, Janet Brandt, Mary Buddemeier, Kenny Cope, Hugh Ferry, Jen Fisette, Connie Fox, Ted France, Marian Franck, Ann Marie Gallo, Jennifer Gorecki, Kim Graber, Tina Hall, Mark Harris, Leslie Hicks, Korey Hill, Christine Hopper, Diedre Jago, Michelle Leising, Stephanie Little, Sue Long, Susan Lynn, Koji Matsushima, Marguerite McDonald, Shauna McGhie, Doug McLeren, Marcia Motz, Diane Mozen, Jamie O'Conner, Karen Pagnano-Richardson, Ben Peasley, Penny Portman, De Raynes, Judy Rink, Gabe Romero, Anne Catherine Sullivan, Phillip Thomas, Julia Valley, Lori Williams, Rachel Williams and Russ Williams.

In addition, NASPE extends its appreciation to more than 100 middle school and high school physical educators, from all across the nation in every type of school and situation, who found time in their limited class hours to administer one or more of the Standards 2-6 cognitive tests. Their participation yielded thousands of student tests, which provided a rich source of data for establishing validity, reliability, item discrimination and other advanced data analysis applications.

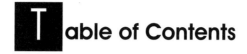

Table of Contents

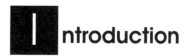

Introduction

Standards-Based Education

Since the late 1980s, education reform in the United States has been driven largely by setting academic standards that describe what students should know and be able to do, and developing accountability systems for measuring student achievement of those standards. Terms such as "standards-based education," "standards-based education reform" and "standards movement" are common in today's education vernacular.

Standards and assessment have been pivotal themes in recent reform efforts, cutting across much of the federal legislation that Congress has passed to improve education for all students. Standards-based education began in 1994, when Congress passed Goals 2000: The Educate America Act. That established a framework for identifying world-class academic standards, measuring student progress and providing support for any student needing help in meeting the standards. Goals 2000 codified eight national education goals:

1. School readiness.

2. School completion.

3. Student achievement & citizenship.

4. Teacher education & professional development.

5. Mathematics and science excellence.

6. Adult literacy & lifelong learning.

7. Alcohol- and drug-free schools.

8. Parental participation.

Since Goals 2000, Congress has twice amended and/or reauthorized the Elementary and Secondary School Education Act of 1965 (ESEA). The 1994 ESEA reauthorization, dubbed the Improving America's Schools Act, focused on changing the way education is delivered, encouraging comprehensive school reform, upgrading instruction and professional development to align with high standards, strengthening accountability and promoting the coordination of resources to improve education for all children.

The most recent ESEA reauthorization, the No Child Left Behind Act of 2001 (NCLB), prescribes increased accountability for states, school districts and schools, greater choice for parents and students (particularly those attending low-performing schools), more flexibility for state and local education agencies in using federal education dollars and a stronger emphasis on reading, especially for the youngest children. Together, those federal laws have established many of the principles of standards-based reform, including the expectation that all students will attain high standards of academic excellence.

Standards-based education requires clear, measurable standards for all students. Standards and benchmarks identify what students should know and be able to do as they progress through school, and should be written so that they are developmentally appropriate and relevant to future education and employment needs. They also should be written so that all students are capable of achieving them, and so that talented students will exceed them.

Standards are meant to be anchors, aligning curriculum, instruction and assessment. That explains the emergence of the terms "standards-based curriculum," "standards-based instruction" and "standards-based assessment," as well as the holistic term "standards-based education." By design, standards-based education lends itself to accountability.

Standards-Based Accountability

In years past, accountability in education was determined by measuring school inputs and processes such as funding levels, curriculum offerings and resources and regulation compliance. After national and state standards emerged, policymakers began to shift the focus of accountability to student outcomes. Now, policymakers emphasize student learning and achievement outcomes to gauge the success of state and local education efforts. This trend in education reform is known as standards-based accountability. Systems have been and continue to be put into place to hold states, districts, schools and teachers accountable for students' performance.

Standards-based accountability systems use criterion-referenced performance standards rather than norm-referenced rankings. A standards-based system measures each student against a concrete standard, instead of measuring how well a student performs when compared to others.

Once standards are established, the next step in building a standards-based accountability system is aligning curriculum to the standards. The knowledge or skills that students must acquire to meet the standards must be defined, and criterion-referenced assessments must be established to determine the extent to which students meet the standards. The alignment of instruction and formative assessment of the standards must follow.

Standards-Based Education & Accountability for Physical Education

The National Association for Sport and Physical Education (NASPE) has established itself as a leader in standards-based education. In 1995, NASPE published *Moving Into the Future: National Standards for Physical Education*, followed by a second edition in 2004.

"Physical activity is critical to the development and maintenance of good health, state NASPE's National Standards. "The goal of physical education is to develop physically educated individuals who have the knowledge, skills and confidence to enjoy a lifetime of healthful physical activity" (NASPE, 2004).

NASPE defines a physically educated person as someone who:

1. Demonstrates competency in motor skills and movement patterns needed to perform a variety of physical activities.

2. Demonstrates understanding of movement concepts, principles, strategies and tactics as they apply to the learning and performance of physical activities.

3. Participates regularly in physical activity.

4. Achieves and maintains a health-enhancing level of physical fitness.

5. Exhibits responsible personal and social behavior that respects self and others in physical activity settings.

6. Values physical activity for health, enjoyment, challenge, self-expression and/or social interaction.

The National Standards are presented in grade-level ranges representing K-2, 3-5, 6-8 and 9-12, so that the ranges are consistent with children's and youths' developmental patterns, that they reflect organizational patterns in public school settings and that they align with other content areas.

Each grade range contains two sections: student expectations and sample performance outcomes. Student expectations reflect what students should know and be able to do at the end of each grade-level range (e.g., grade 8). Sample performance outcomes are examples of student behavior at each grade-level range that demonstrate progress toward meeting the standards.

Until now, nationally tested assessments and rubrics to measure student achievement of the National Standards and benchmarks have been the missing elements of standards-based physical education. With the publication of PE Metrics for elementary, now followed by PE Metrics for middle and high school, NASPE has closed the gap.

PE Metrics provides valid and reliable standards-based assessments and rubrics ("NASPE assessments") to measure student achievement of the National Standards by high school graduation and appropriate progress at four other grade-level ranges. The assessments in this book give evidence of learning through student work/performance, and their rubrics describe the quality of the work/performance. With PE Metrics, teachers and schools have the ability to report student progress on each standard. The advantage to that approach is that it provides students, teachers and parents with highly specific information.

It's critical to align curriculum, instruction and assessments with one another and with state and national standards. To provide students with a truly standards-based physical education, teachers must be certain that the material on which students are being assessed aligns with what's being taught in class.

Assessment as part of the instruction process constitutes much more than evaluation and accountability. Teachers should use a variety of techniques, including NASPE assessments, as part of regular classroom instruction. Assessment integrated with instruction (e.g., pre-assessment and formative assessment) is imperative for maximizing student learning and success. It's equally important to use pre-assessment and formative assessment to communicate important skills and knowledge to students and to prepare students properly for summative assessment.

For accountability purposes, it isn't necessary to assess all students on every task; one can use a random sample of student performance to guide curriculum development and/or to report on programmatic success to school, district and/or state leaders.

Whether one uses PE Metrics assessments as part of the instruction process (e.g., pre-assessment and formative assessment) or for evaluation and accountability, they are scientifically valid and useful tools for measuring student achievement.

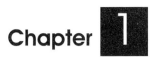

Chapter 1

Overview of NASPE's PE Metrics Assessment Project

The National Association for Sport and Physical Education (NASPE) is committed to the tenets of high-quality physical education, which include the opportunity for all students to learn through supportive policies and environment (e.g., certified teachers, adequate facilities and equipment), National Standards, high-quality curriculum, appropriate instruction practices, and student and program assessment. NASPE continues to develop tools to help schools, districts and states implement assessments that measure student progress toward state and national physical education standards. As the only national association for physical education, NASPE feels a strong obligation to develop valid and reliable assessments that teachers throughout the nation can use.

In March 1999, NASPE assembled a "think tank" of university and public school professionals to consider how to best advance K-12 physical education. The group was charged with recommending a plan of action to confront the barriers to high-quality physical education. The priority recommendation was to develop performance indicators and practical assessments to evaluate student progress toward the National Standards for Physical Education.

In January 2000, NASPE created what became known as its Assessment Task Force, made up of experts in curriculum and instruction and measurement and evaluation, researchers, teacher educators, K-12 physical education teachers, administrators and students. NASPE charged the task force with developing performance indicators that corresponded to the National Standards at each grade-level range (K-2, 3-5, 6-8 and 9-12), as well as assessments for each indicator. The performance indicators were not meant to be a comprehensive set of all possible skills and knowledge that students should master in a specific grade-level range, but rather samples of performance outcomes that could be expected within that grade-level range.

Performance Indicators & Assessment Development

Just as it was not feasible to identify all possible performance indicators, it became clear to the task force that it would not be feasible to write all possible assessments for each indicator. Ultimately, the task force identified a broad range of performance indicators and wrote a variety of assessments to measure student skills and knowledge. The examples selected and presented in this book and CD-ROM provide templates of good assessments that can serve to guide teachers, districts and states in developing additional assessments.

Standard 1

Initially, task force members were paired with content experts, and writing the assessments occurred over a period of several years. The draft performance indicators and assessments that they developed were introduced to 220 professionals attending a session at the 2001 American Alliance for Health, Physical Education, Recreation and Dance (AAHPERD) National Convention. NASPE continued to revise the indicators and assessments and to solicit member feedback during the development stages at AAHPERD National Conventions each year, as well as at other state and regional conferences.

Standards 2-6

Once the Standard 1 assessments were written and in the process of being pilot-tested, the task force focused on developing assessments for Standards 2-6. After writing performance indicators, the task force originally developed a series of authentic assessments for Standards 2-6. As early drafts of the assessments were tested, however, it became clear that the task force would not be able to develop authentic assessments (e.g., determining student ability to cooperate in class) that were reliable and valid. Therefore, the task force decided to use written tests (multiple-choice) to measure learning outcomes for Standards 2-6. These tests were written by small committees of content experts, under the direction of task force members.

The test-writing committees developed tables of specifications to ensure that the questions were written at the appropriate level of difficulty and reading comprehension and were linked to the content within each performance indicator. Rather than developing five separate tests (one for each standard), the committees grouped the questions into three broad concept areas (Standard 2; Standards 3 & 4; and Standards 5 & 6). The committees wrote three forms (A, B & C), with 40 multiple-choice items each for the grade 8 and high school levels.

Institutional Review Board Approval

In preparing for the data collection, NASPE obtained Institutional Review Board (IRB) approval for using human subjects in a research study from the University of Illinois at Urbana-Champaign (UIUC) and Northern Illinois University (NIU). NASPE obtained IRB approval in 2003, and it has been renewed each year. Although the IRB document was written to enable project administrators from different universities to use the same consent documents, the project administrators were advised to make sure that UIUC's IRB approval would satisfy the IRB requirements at their home institutions. In the end, all project administrators submitted joint agreements with UIUC or were covered under NIU's IRB. NASPE obtained an additional IRB from NIU for administering Standards 2-6 tests.

Following data collection for the elementary project, NIU granted an IRB exemption for the Standards 2-6 multiple-choice tests for the national data collection, because of the nature of the anonymous multiple-choice test format and because these types of assessments are commonly conducted in physical education classes.

Data Collectors

Standard 1

NASPE trained teacher educators to supervise the administration of the pilot and national data collection for Standard 1. These project administrators were chosen based on four criteria:

1. They had established contacts with teachers and administrators in the public schools through their placements of pre-service students for field experience.

2. They had experience with video-recording student performances.

3. They had knowledge of the appropriate execution of motor skills.

4. Their research backgrounds meant that they understood the importance of adhering strictly to testing protocols, including obtaining school district permission and parent/student consent for testing, as well as following the exact assessment description and instructions, including equipment, site preparation, safety and video-recording.

Project administrators were recruited through personal contacts made by NASPE staff and task force members. They received six hours of training that included a project history and overview, roles and responsibilities (including gaining entry, informed consent, video-recording and coding), protocols for video-recording and conducting the assessments, typical video-recording problems and guidelines for coding the video records. Training took place at AAHPERD National Conventions (2004, 2005, 2006 & 2007) and at regional and district conferences (2004, 2007).

Standards 2-6

Task force members and NASPE staff recruited secondary physical education teachers from around the country to administer the tests to their students. The tests, detailed instructions, consent forms and Scantron answer sheets were sent to the teachers and subsequently returned to the researcher at NIU for initial analysis. In addition to administering the tests, teachers were asked to review questions for content and readability and to provide feedback to the task force.

Process for Testing & Data Collection

Standard 1 assessments and Standards 2-6 written tests were subjected to the following sequence of testing:

- Pre-pilot data collection.

- Pilot data collection.

- National data collection.

Because Standard 1 measures skill performance, testing involved video-recording each assessment, then coding the videos to produce scores for each aspect of students' performance. Because of the seasonal nature of instruction in physical education (e.g., restrictions imposed by inclement weather, some units taught only in the spring or fall), pilot and national data collection took longer than anticipated. Because Standards 2-6 assessments are paper-and-pencil tests that measure students' cognitive knowledge, they were easier to administer, required fewer personnel and were completed more quickly than the Standard 1 assessments.

Pre-Pilot Data Collection

Standard 1

All assessments were pre-piloted by at least one secondary teacher and 20 students. Teachers provided feedback on the instructions to teachers and students, camera placement and level of difficulty for the assessment task. The task force revised the assessments based on that feedback, as well as on feedback obtained during AAHPERD National Convention sessions. During the pre-pilot phase, NASPE reduced the number of National Standards from seven to six. As a result, in 2005, the task force modified both the performance indicators and assessments to meet the new standards and grade-level ranges. Accordingly, the task force collected additional data and pre-pilot feedback for some of the Standard 1 assessments.

Standards 2-6

Three forms of each test at each grade level were administered to a minimum of 20 students in December 2008, and teachers provided feedback on readability, clarity and ease of administration. The task force revised questions based on teacher feedback and on conventional data analysis (item difficulty and discrimination). Based on the analysis, the task force identified the 10 strongest questions, which were used as common questions on each form of the three tests (A, B & C) to be used for pilot testing.

Pilot Data Collection

Standard 1

Project administrators subsequently tested the assessments on a larger scale to further ensure their appropriateness and to collect preliminary data on discrimination, validity and reliability. The task force collected data from various sections of the country through an extensive network of project administrators.

At least 40 students completed each pilot assessment. Project administrators collected parent/student/teacher consent forms, worked with a secondary physical education teacher to administer the assessments and video-recorded, coded and provided feedback on the assessments. The data were analyzed to ensure that the assessments were appropriately difficult and that they revealed meaningful differences among students. The task force revised the assessments as needed, based on data analysis and the feedback from teachers and project administrators.

Standards 2-6

The task force and NASPE staff recruited teachers from around the United States at AAHPERD and district conventions, and from personal contacts to conduct one or more cognitive assessments, and 200 students completed each of the three forms of the Standards 2-6 test in January and February 2009. Data analysis identified a problem with discrimination and difficulty levels with a number of questions, so the task force revised the problematic questions. All the questions were pilot-tested again in October 2009 with a smaller number of students. The resulting data were analyzed, and the best questions were used to create two forms (A & B) of the test for each grade level for the national data collection.

National Data Collection

Standard 1

Data collection for the Standard 1 assessments began in February 2005 and continued through spring 2010. (The IRB approval from UIUC continued to cover national data collection.) NASPE requested an additional IRB, which NIU approved each year from 2007 to 2010 to cover a subset of data collectors not named originally in the UIUC IRB. (See Table 1 on p. 27 for the list of assessments for which national data were collected.)

The project administrators' goal was to collect data from a minimum of 200 students for every assessment task. Two common tasks of medium difficulty were identified at each grade-level range, and students at each grade-level range completed at least one of the two common tasks. The common tasks for Standard 1 secondary assessments were:

- Grade 8: soccer 3 on 2 and volleyball.
- High School: volleyball and weight training.

The data from the common tasks were used in the research process to allow scores to be placed on a common scale. A common scale is important for being able to equate assessments across and within grade-level ranges and to create an assessment bank. These topics are explored further in the Psychometric Quality of Assessments chapter.

Standards 2-6

National data collection for the secondary grade levels occurred in spring 2010, with 400 students completing each form of the test (A & B) at each grade level (grade 8 and high school). Data analysis was conducted in June 2010.

Summary

NASPE's Assessment Task Force has followed a long and difficult path in creating the PE Metrics assessments. In all, the process took more than 10 years of concerted, ongoing effort by the entire task force and writing team members. Task force members believe that this careful and extensive process has resulted in valid and reliable assessments that are useful for teachers, administrators, teacher educators and researchers in both physical education and the wider field of education in general. The task force views its work as a first step in NASPE's ongoing effort to create and then add to a body of assessments for our field.

Chapter 2

Using PE Metrics Assessments

In today's education climate, there's no place in the school curriculum for a program area that can neither define the outcomes that students should achieve nor measure the extent to which they have met those outcomes. Too many physical education programs have largely avoided doing both. The instruction process is said to be one of planning or defining outcomes, teaching so that students achieve those outcomes and assessing the extent to which students have mastered those outcomes. Too often, physical educators have felt that assessment "takes time away from instruction," and they have failed to recognize that assessment is a critical part of effective instruction.

The National Standards for Physical Education provide a guide for determining the critical outcomes of physical education. The standards articulate exit outcomes for the K-12 program. Effective physical education programs must measure student performance at particular grade levels en route to attaining the standards. The PE Metrics assessment materials provide grade-level performance indicators and related assessments that are valid and reliable measures to help with this process.

The assessment materials in this book were not designed to measure all program outcomes related to the National Standards but rather to identify critical outcomes in specific content areas at particular grade levels. They are not a "test" but are, rather, a resource of assessment materials that teachers and administrators can put together to meet the needs of particular programs. The number of rubrics for Standard 1 activities is most certainly not a comprehensive set of the activities taught by most schools but do provide a sampling of different types of activities that should be a part of good secondary program. (NASPE might develop rubrics for additional activities in the future.)

Assessment materials should match what is taught in a program. Therefore, NASPE encourages professionals at all levels to select the assessments that are appropriate for their programs' goals.

Using the Assessments in This Book

The assessment materials in this book, in the accompanying CD-ROM and on the PE Metrics Web site, www.PEMetrics.org, are intended for use at different levels for a variety of purposes. Teachers; schools; school district administrators; local, state and national policymakers; and researchers will find them useful in different ways.

1. Teachers

The PE Metrics program is a total package that provides teachers with assessment materials that they can use in a variety of ways. It's also a package that provides teachers with a way to interpret and report assessment.

Using PE Metrics for Formative & Summative Assessment

Teachers use both formative and summative assessment as part of the instruction process. The assessment materials in this book facilitate both types of assessment. Standard 1 (motor skills) is measured using observation rubrics that will be useful for both formative and summative assessment. Standards 2-6 assessments are written test items — provided both in this book in print form and on the accompanying CD-ROM — that teachers can use as formative or summative assessments.

Formative assessment helps teachers determine students' skill levels before and during the instruction phase. It's easy for teachers to make inaccurate assumptions about students' abilities when planning a unit of instruction, so testing them before planning the unit can make instruction far more appropriate.

Assessing students before planning a unit allows teachers to compare the results of assessment conducted prior to the unit with that conducted at the end of the unit (summative assessment). This practice — often referred to as pre- and post-assessment — facilitates teachers' ability to determine how much students have learned from instruction. Teachers can use the Standard 1 rubrics in this book to pre- and post-test students. They also can consider selecting items from the Standards 2-6 test bank provided on the CD-ROM as a pretest of what a student knows at the beginning of the school year.

Teachers also can use the Standard 1 rubrics to track students' performance over time, and to help students track their own performance. The newest motivation theories stress the importance of assessing students on their improvement over time and establishing learning climates that are mastery-oriented (students work for personal improvement) rather than ego-oriented (students are focused on comparing themselves to others).

The rubrics provided in this book can enable secondary students to conduct peer and self-assessments, as well as helping them set goals. Assessment data can help students set appropriate goals and track progress toward those goals. Using peer or self-assessment during the instruction process can motivate students to do well and helps provide them with a clear understanding of performance expectations, particularly when used in conjunction with personal goal-setting.

Summative assessment helps teachers identify how much students have learned as a result of instruction. Summative assessment occurs at the end of the instruction process. Valid and reliable assessment tools are critical to summative assessment. Teachers should use valid and reliable assessments to determine the effectiveness of instruction and student grades. Reports sent to parents and policymakers on student achievement should be based on objective data. The PE Metrics assessments are ideally suited for these purposes, because they're targeted toward the outcomes of instruction that is appropriate for different grade-level ranges.

While teachers can use the Standard 1 rubrics in this book to assess students on multiple occasions during the instruction process, they can't use the written multiple choice test items designed for Standards 2-6 for that purpose without jeopardizing their value as a summative measure. Two sets of the written test items are available. The first set is provided in this book and on the accompanying CD-ROM, and can be used formatively. The second set is available only with PE Metrics Online — NASPE's Web-based service that allows teachers, schools and school districts to track student performance over time and to generate reports for parents and administrators (visit PEMetrics.org) — and should be used as a summative measure of student knowledge in Standards 2-6.

Sampling Students to Collect Assessment Data

NASPE designed its PE Metrics Standard 1 assessments so that each assessment has a difficulty level. This means that teachers can conduct different assessments with different students and still equate the performance between the students. They also can assess different classes of the same grade on different assessments, compare scores and not have to assess every class on every assessment.

Using PE Metrics for Formative Assessment

Teachers will agree that the skills and strategies assessed through PE Metrics are not equally difficult. Indeed, a score of a 4 on a relatively simple task should not lead you to expect that the student would score a 4 on a more difficult task. The fact that not all teachers teach the same skills and strategies at the same time can lead to uneven comparison of students. If you taught a unit that involved a simple skill, and your colleague taught a more difficult skill, comparing PE Metrics assessments from your classes might lead to an erroneous conclusion that your students — with higher assessment scores — are better performers.

The issue is that a 4 on one rubric is not necessarily equal to a 4 on another, and it might even equal a 2 on another. Because PE Metrics was created using Item Response Theory, this unevenness can be accounted for by creating an ability score. The ability score allows teachers to compare scores from each rubric to scores from other rubrics in the book. Those scores are calibrated by difficulty.

Calculating students' ability scores will reflect each assessment's actual difficulty for the purpose of estimating a student's ability overall. Scores on different rubrics should not be compared and cannot be equated, but ability scores can. You can calculate ability scores using the Ability Score Calculator found at www.PEMetrics.org. Simply enter each student's raw score, by dimension, and the tool will calculate the student's ability score.

Ability scores are most useful as formative information. Let's say that you're teaching content for which you can use two PE Metrics assessments to provide information on student learning. For example, in an eighth-grade class, you taught soccer and administered the soccer 3-on-2 assessment at the end of the unit. You followed your soccer unit with the team handball unit and, at the end of that unit, you used the team handball 3-on-2 assessment.

Chris, one of your students, recorded scores of 3 on each dimension of each assessment rubric. Therefore, Chris is competent in each of the assessment tasks. But you are more interested in Chris's true ability in regard to Standard 1, so you must convert Chris's rubric scores to ability scores on each assessment. Using the Ability Score Calculator, you find that Chris earned one ability score on the soccer assessment and earned a higher ability score on the team handball assessment. Because Chris's ability scores increased, you can say with confidence that Chris has improved, is learning and, ultimately, has achieved competence in the standard. *Note:* You need not have repeated the soccer 3-v-2 assessment to learn that Chris had achieved competence in regard to Standard 1.

Using PE Metrics for Grading

In addition to PE Metrics' formative use, teachers often will wish to use it as a summative assessment, for grading. We understand that teachers need a valid and reliable set of tools to calculate grades, and the Standard 1 assessments in this book use a four-point rubric, which might tempt some readers to translate those scores into a four-point grade scale, in which 4 = A, 3 = B, etc. That is not an appropriate use of this tool.

As a summative assessment, it's appropriate to use PE Metrics to determine the extent to which a student has met competence for Standard 1. Teachers don't need to average ability scores to do that. An average ability score is virtually meaningless; it's the final ability score that determines the student's level of competence. Therefore, if administering the two assessments, as in the example above, Chris earned two scores, you could take the higher and use it for a grade. *Remember:* It's not the actual raw scores from the assessment rubrics that hold meaning for grading purposes, but the calculation of ability scores.

To use ability scores as grades, teachers must be clear about grade standards. It's necessary to understand that demonstrating competence (a score of 3 or 4) does not mean that the student is competent in Standard 1. For example, a student scoring a 3 ("competent") on a simple assessment might have an ability score of 230. Therefore, while the student demonstrated competence on this particular assessment, he/she has not yet attained competence on Standard 1 for that grade level. The student must attain an ability score of 500 (on any assessment) to demonstrate competence on Standard 1.

If grading is your intention with PE Metrics ability scores, you'll need to develop a scoring rubric in which ability scores are converted to letter grades. It's not the intent of this publication to develop such a rubric, as grades are the purview of individual teachers or schools.

If you're converting assessment scores to ability scores, it's important to use the highest ability score, not the average of the ability scores, regardless of the assessment task, to compute ability, then convert to grades.

Ideally, teachers will construct grades to reflect students' achievement of learning objectives. Certainly, developing skills, strategies and abilities in games and activities, achieving fitness, and enhancing personal and social responsibility are goals of most physical education programs, and grades reflecting students' achievement of objectives related to those goals are appropriate.

Teachers might have specific learning objectives that reflect tasks measured by the PE Metrics assessments. It's reasonable to state learning objectives for students to be able to play a modified game of touch football, for example, or to demonstrate a golf pre-swing stance, full swing, chip and putt. Teachers must remember, however, that the purpose of the PE Metrics Standard 1 assessments is to assess competence within Standard 1. Grades include many factors, some of which are not related to competence within Standard 1. Competence in a modified game of touch football is not a goal; it's an objective that will lead to the goal of competence within Standard 1.

Teachers can consider students' achievement of standards when grading, but that information is used more appropriately at a classroom, school or district level, announced as a percentage of students who have achieved the standard.

Reports to Parents

Using PE Metrics will allow teachers to compile data in different forms and send reports on student achievement to parents and guardians with suggestions for how they can help their children improve.

Teacher Preparation for Using PE Metrics Materials

Although teachers can use PE Metrics both formally and informally, the materials were designed as formal assessments. This means that if teachers want to compare student scores, the assessments have to be conducted according to the procedures provided. That's sometimes difficult for teachers who might want to improvise the space or equipment used, or who want to coach students differently about how to complete an assessment. To use the materials in this book appropriately, teachers must attend to the procedures provided, which requires preparation. That involves learning how to administer the test items and how to score them, which is explored in the next chapter.

2. District Administrators

PE Metrics assessment materials have many potential uses at the school district level. A district can more effectively help students meet physical education standards by graduation if it uses assessment data to track students' progress as they move through the K-12 program. For example, elementary, middle and high school programs can become better aligned with one another, and districts can standardize expectations for students across grades and schools. Used that way, assessment can help districts improve their curriculum planning.

Many physical education programs have functioned without accountability for student learning because there has been no systematic way to measure teacher effectiveness and little effort to measure student performance. Accountability does not limit good programs and teachers; rather, it enhances them. With accountability systems in place, schools can provide students with feedback on their level of performance and learning, and can provide parents with information about their children's progress. Assessment data allows schools and districts to track student achievement, evaluate curriculum needs and promote program improvement.

Districts don't need assessment data on each student to evaluate programs. Classes can be sampled to provide a measure of program assessment. Because NASPE developed PE Metrics assessments with a difficulty score for each assessment, districts can compare schools using different assessments.

Through assessment and accountability, physical education takes its place as a critical part of the overall school program. On the other hand, a lack of accountability can protect poor programs and ineffective teachers. Districts will find valid and reliable assessments essential to conducting high-quality physical education programs that produce graduates who value physical activity and have the knowledge and skills to be physically active adults.

3. Local, State & National Policymakers

Consciously or subconsciously, physical educators often overstate what their programs do for students. The field of physical education has claimed much but provided little evidence that it can deliver on these promises to students. Policymakers at all levels want to know whether the resources they pour into any program have any impact on students. Physical education programs in some areas of the country have been cut recently to provide more time for other academic subjects. Without valid assessment data, it's difficult to advocate that physical education programs can exert an impact on both the traditional goals of our programs and current national health problems.

With PE Metrics assessment materials, though, policymakers will have tools to determine the impact of physical education programs, assess student knowledge and skills in terms of program goals, track student progress over time, compare program quality across districts and states, and provide a way to hold teachers, schools, districts and states responsible for assessing outcomes and meeting program goals.

4. Researchers

Research on curriculum and instruction in physical education has been hampered by a lack of valid and reliable tools to assess student outcomes. A considerable amount of the research conducted on teaching, teachers and curriculum in physical education has been related to the processes of teaching without attending to the products of those processes. It's critical that the physical education profession be able to identify how to provide students with the skills, knowledge and dispositions they need to lead a physically active lifestyle. Evidence-based practice depends on good research, and good research depends on having a valid and reliable way to measure student achievement.

Valid outcome measures enable us to answer these questions:

- To what extent are the National Standards being achieved?

- Are students who achieve more related to the National Standards more physically active than those who achieve less?

- What curricula are most effective in helping students to achieve the national standards, and under what conditions for what outcomes?

- How do the standards relate to one another? For example, what is the relationship of skill in movement forms to participation in physical activity and fitness levels? How do we instruct students effectively to meet the outcomes we target?

- How are good physical education programs related to academic achievement?

The answers to those questions depend on having good measures of student performance. The PE Metrics assessment materials provide a foundation for measurement, data collection over time and accountability.

Misusing Assessment

Although assessment is a powerful tool for improving instruction and learning, it carries the potential for unintended and negative consequences. Assessment is being misused when:

- Students are assessed on concepts and skills that they haven't been taught or haven't been given enough time to learn.

- What's being assessed becomes the whole curriculum rather than a measured sample of what students should be learning as a part of a comprehensive curriculum.

- Scores that students receive on assessments are used exclusively to evaluate students, teachers, schools, districts or states.

- Using raw scores from different rubrics to compare students. Grades should be calculated from ability scores.

While the PE Metrics assessments target critical outcomes that all students should achieve, they are not the only important outcomes of a good program. The ultimate goal in PE Metrics is to improve the quality of physical education programs. The assessment materials in this book can provide teachers, students, parents, administrators and policymakers with both formative and summative data. That information helps teachers improve instruction and demonstrate student learning. Administrators and policymakers also can use the data to determine the impact of physical education programs and, subsequently, to support those programs.

A Note About Some of the Scoring Rubrics

Several of the Standard 1 middle school scoring rubrics (softball, pickleball, floor hockey and folk dance) did not yield sufficient samples to ensure accurate ability scores. They are still useful assessments, but any ability score that users compile for them might not be accurate.

Likewise, wall climbing and flag football at the high school level might yield inaccurate ability scores, and users cannot calculate an ability score for high school bowling and tennis at this time. NASPE will make every effort to increase the sample size for those activities so that readers can use them to calculate ability scores. In the meantime, though, readers should consider these rubrics effective assessment tools for all other purposes.

A note appears at the top of the first page of those scoring rubrics indicating their status.

Chapter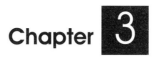

Administering & Scoring PE Metrics Assessments

Standard 1

As part of the research procedures for this project, NASPE's Assessment Task Force collected data according to a rubric connected to each Standard 1 assessment. All student performances were video-recorded to facilitate data analysis, which included intra- and inter-rater reliability coding for data collection. Thousands of students participated in the national sample and provided data. The results of the coding enabled the task force to improve the quality and clarity of individual assessments and determine the most effective testing protocols.

For teachers using the PE Metrics assessments, video-recording allows them to view student performance on more than one occasion. It also enables greater scoring accuracy, because teachers can conduct an "instant replay" of an assessment by simply reviewing all or part of the record. Many of the secondary assessments are complex game-play situations, and it's very difficult to score students without a video-recording that one can replay to review individual student performance. Video-recording also provides teachers with hard evidence for documenting student achievement. Finally, video records provide a mechanism for teachers to conduct periodic self-checks of their scoring reliability.

This section of this book contains procedures and directions for administering the assessments. The procedures and directions guide standardized administration of the assessments. Teachers who are conducting summative assessments must follow the procedures in each assessment precisely so that they can compare performances later, pre- and post-test, class to class, year to year, teacher to teacher or school to school. Before using the assessments (with the exception of pre-assessment), teachers should ensure that students have been taught the task and have had numerous opportunities to practice the skills exactly as described in the assessment.

Remember: Follow school or district guidelines regarding permission to record student performances.

Procedures for Administering the Assessments & Collecting Data
Administering the Assessments

Standard 1
Preparation
1. Prepare the score sheets ahead of time and have pencils, clipboard, stopwatch and other activity equipment required for the assessment on site.
2. Prepare all equipment (and, perhaps, some spare equipment) before the class enters the assessment setting. This should include taping mats, inflating balls, distributing safety mats and removing objects/equipment from around the perimeter of the space.
3. Prepare alternative activities for students who are not involved in the assessments. Ensure that they're active, supervised and safe.
4. Once the assessment area is identified and marked, set up the camera and record a trial run of the assessment before class to ensure that the viewfinder can "see" all essential elements of the entire assessment.

Video-Recording

1. When movement in rhythm to an accompaniment is part of the assessment, place camera and music source (if used) close together so that you can hear the music later, when reviewing the video record.

2. Camera set-up directions for each assessment are provided in the individual assessments. Follow them for each assessment unless your testing situation requires a different set-up. Ultimately, you must be able to see the entire activity area needed for an assessment, the trajectory or path of the ball or implement, the target when indicated, and the student's entire body (e.g., feet, head). That might require moving some cameras back farther if they don't have wide-angle lenses. It also might require adjusting the angle for the situation.

Safety Considerations

1. The court or floor surface should be dry, clean and clear of obstacles surrounding and beyond the boundary of the test area. Adequate out-of-bounds space is important for deceleration and turning, etc.

2. If you're assessing outdoors, ensure that the surface is appropriate. A hard surface should be dry, smooth and clean. If the assessment calls for a grassy area, it should be mowed and free of grass clippings, hazards, trash, holes and obstructions.

3. Allow only safe footwear; no sandals, boots or bare feet.

4. Ensure that students know the testing area boundaries, that they understand the markings, are aware of the deceleration or stopping zone, and are clear about their personal space.

5. Set up the testing area so that other students can't enter it inadvertently.

6. Have students performing the assessment face away from distractions during testing.

7. Have students empty their pockets, remove jewelry, tie their shoes and take off accessories that might injure them or a partner. This is especially important for assessments that require rolling or inverted positions and/or performance with or against another person.

Warm-Up & Practice

1. A warm-up and short practice period is recommended. The assessments shouldn't be a secret; students should have had adequate learning time in previous lessons.

2. Don't recite directions to a dance during the assessment, and don't use music that has the directions on it.

Test Administration

1. As noted above, follow the camera set-up and placement directions for each assessment.

2. If possible, have a teacher administer the assessment and have another person record the performance.

3. Read "Directions to Students" exactly as they're written, so that the directions are audible to the students and on the video recording.

4. Be sure that all students understand the directions. Read them to the entire class. Teachers might need to reread the instructions periodically if a long period of time elapses after having read them initially. Be fair; if it makes sense to read the instructions again for a student, do so.

5. Don't permit other students to act as an audience for those being assessed; make arrangements for others to be physically active and adequately supervised.

6. Ensure that the order of the students on the code sheet matches the order of the students on the video record. Record student names as seen on the video on the code sheet.

7. If feasible, have each student say his/her name in front of the camera in a loud voice immediately before beginning the assessment. Ask each student to stand 5 feet (sufficient distance to see the student's body) in front of the camera and state his/her name clearly. Alternatively, the assistant recording the assessment could say the student's name.

8. Use a "Ready/Start" signal to begin the assessment.

9. Be sure that students know what to do if action stops, whether they can restart and what to do if the ball goes far out of bounds. Also, be sure that they:

   a. Understand the important elements of an assessment (e.g., they might think that speed is the critical element, when the critical elements are accurate passes and controlling receptions).

   b. Understand that they should resume an interrupted skill during a timed assessment.

Coding Protocols

Study the assessment

1. Read the entire assessment carefully.

2. Study the major focus of each criterion.

3. Study the value difference of each level for all criteria, noting that Level 3 equals competence.

Preview/view the video record before trying to score

1. Look for the major focus of each criterion (practice for recognition of each).

2. Look for the differences in performance in relation to the quality level of each criterion (range of proficiency among performers; common errors).

3. Become familiar with the requirements of the criteria and corresponding performance levels of the assessments. A Level 4 performance should be effortless, refined and performed without hesitation. Typically, only a very small number of students in each class will be able to demonstrate a Level 4 performance.

Practice Scoring

1. View the first performer and make a decision about the first criterion and then all of the other criteria.

2. View as many times as necessary until you can determine a score consistently on each viewing.

3. Focus on one student at a time when the performance includes multiple students (dance, game situations), repeating the above steps for each.

4. Repeat until all students in the performance have been scored on all criteria.

Scoring (Use score sheet designed for each assessment)

1. Record student name and gender.

2. Record scores for all criteria and trials and for all students, as the assessment requires.

3. Total the scores for all criteria and record them on the score sheet in the designated column.

4. Repeat steps above for all performers on the video record.

Scoring Sheet Information

1. Fill out all of the scoring sheets for future use.

2. On the cover of the DVD or tape that you've used for the video record, write the school name and location (to prevent confusion should the DVD become separated from the cover).

Standards 2-6

Administering the Standards 2-6 assessments is considerably easier than administering the Standard 1 assessments, because they're written multiple-choice tests. Administer and score the tests as you would any written test. Find a quiet place and provide students with pencils and the test forms. If possible, use a classroom, so that students can use desks.

This book and the accompanying CD-ROM provide the questions, divided by performance descriptor so that you can select questions based on the content you've taught the students. If you want to assess only a few weeks' worth of instruction, five questions might cover the material. If you are assessing a larger amount of content, you can select more questions. The questions on the CD-ROM are ready for you to cut and paste into a test for students. The answer key is at the end of the questions. In the printed version of the test questions in this book, the correct answers are in **bold** type.

Chapter 4

Psychometric Quality of Assessments

The assessments developed based on the National Standards for Physical Education must be psychometrically sound to make valid and reliable inferences of a student's ability. This chapter first provides a brief description of some key measurement concepts and theories employed in the PE Metrics project; namely, an assessment bank, item response theory and test equating. The chapter then describes calibrations of the assessments for Standards 1 and 2-6. Calibration is a process that sets assessment tasks on a common measurement scale and determines their psychometric quality.

New Concepts, Theory & Techniques Employed
Online Bank of Assessments

In addition to publishing the assessment materials in book form, NASPE is developing an online bank of physical education assessments that share the same scale and that teachers will be able to access easily to select tasks tailored to a specific group of students. This bank of assessments — parts of which readers can access by visiting www.PEMetrics.org — includes Standard 1 assessments ranked for difficulty that allow teachers to select appropriately difficult tasks for a student or class of students, as well as Standards 2-6 cognitive assessments.

Building an assessment bank depends heavily on two major new advances in modern assessment practice:

1. Item Response Theory.
2. Test equating.

Item Response Theory (IRT)

IRT was developed during the 1950s and 1960s in education measurement practice. Its relatively slow development accelerated in the 1980s due to the growing accessibility of personal computers and development of application software. Today, IRT is the most dominant theory for test construction within all major testing organizations and agencies.

When compared to measurement models based on the classical test theory, which has been the primary testing theory in the field of physical education, models based upon IRT have several advantages (Hambleton, Swaminathan & Rogers, 1991; Spray, 1987). The primary advantages of IRT are that item parameters are independent of the ability level of the examinees responding to the items; and, at the same time, the ability parameters are independent of the items used in tests and the performance of other examinees. This is known as IRT's "invariance" feature. That is, the assessment item is not tied to the ability of the student, and the students are not bound to the difficulty of the test.

Because of that feature, interpreting item difficulty and examinee ability is consistent in IRT. For example, a difficult item will not become easier when it's applied to a group of examinees with higher abilities.

Another important advantage of IRT is that item difficulty and student ability are set on the same scale, which makes it much easier to determine the appropriateness of an item for a given ability level and to interpret test scores. As a result, a teacher can select an assessment that is appropriately difficult for a student and can explain what the student's score really means. IRT has been used in physical education for many years and has been well-tested for its measurement advantages. (See Safrit, Zhu, Costa & Zhang, 1992; Spray, 1987; Zhu, 1996, 2006; Zhu & Cole, 1996; Zhu & Safrit, 1993; for more information.)

Test Equating

Test equating is a statistical procedure used to establish the relationship between scores from two or more tests or to place them on a common scale. The task of equating, in general, is to establish statistically a conversion relationship among summary scores from two or more test forms or tests. The relationship could be linear or non-linear, depending on the equating method employed.

Test-equating methods, according to the test theory on which they are based, generally can be classified into two categories: traditional and IRT (Kolen & Brennan, 2004; Zhu, 1998). With test equating, putting two or more tests on the same scale becomes possible, which is also necessary for establishing an item or assessment bank.

A number of successful test-equating applications in fitness testing based upon traditional equating approaches have been reported (Zhu, 1998, 2001). As a result, teachers can select any one assessment and will be able to anticipate a student's performance accurately on a different and dissimilar assessment. In this case, test equating will allow a comparison between a group of students' abilities in a basketball unit with a different group of students' abilities in a soccer unit.

A bank of Standard 1 assessments can provide several advantages for teachers and data collectors. First, because the assessment tasks are set on the same scale, testing scores generated will be equivalent to each other even when a different task is assessed. That allows cross-school comparison even when different tasks are used.

In the past, cross-school comparisons often were established by using raw scores, rather than scaled scores. As a result, student performances often depended on the difficulties of the assessments selected, making it very difficult to achieve objective cross-comparisons. For example, one school doing pull-ups and one doing modified pull-ups previously could not be compared. With scaled scores, the difficulty of an assessment is taken into consideration for the scaling process. Therefore, kindergarten students in the first-period class who completed the hopping assessment can be compared to students in the second-period class who completed the striking assessment.

Note: Because no linking items were administered in the middle and high school assessments contained within this book, readers cannot compare assessments across those grade levels. Readers can, however, compare two assessments within a grade level — high school archery and swimming, for example — because they were set on the same scale.

Second, because the difficulty of each item in this set of assessments is known, and the discrimination ability between items is known, teachers can select Standard 1 assessment tasks that target specific levels of student learning. For example, a set of tasks usually is administered to all students; however, very difficult or easy items usually do not work well for students at low or high ends of the ability scale, since these students either all score at the top (a Level 4 performance) or at the bottom (Level 1). If that is the case, then the assessment has failed to discriminate and is generally ineffective at providing information about ability.

With PE Metrics' bank of Standard 1 assessments, teachers can select assessments with appropriate difficulties for a targeted group. This selection process, known as computerized adaptive testing, can make student assessment very time-efficient. Teachers can select appropriately difficult assessments for each student, even though the assessments are different. While this aspect of the assessment bank might not be particularly useful when the goal is to assess basketball skills, it's tremendously useful if the goal is to assess competence within Standard 1.

Think of the process in this way: Suppose that you want to determine a student's upper-body strength and use a pull-up test as the assessment. You would see a lot of "0" scores, because the test was too difficult. A push-up assessment, on the other hand, would yield far fewer "0" scores, and the range of scores would be wider. Unless you have established a link between the two assessments, you would have no way to equate a score of one pull-up to a score of five push-ups.

Additionally, if a push-up assessment is too problematic to administer, the teacher might create a bench-press-type assessment. Scores on that assessment would not be linked to either test, but could be linked then compared via this process. The process used in the PE Metrics assessment project one day will allow teachers and researchers to equate different scores across students.

Finally, an assessment bank makes possible an accurate assessment of student change or growth. Previously, when it became obvious that a task was either too difficult or too easy for a student or groups of students, a different test was developed for them. The problem with that procedure is that the "new" test was not related to the original one, and teachers had no way to determine what a student's ability would be on the original test.

An assessment bank can eliminate that problem because the scores will be equivalent, even if they are generated from different tasks.

As NASPE develops the PE Metrics assessment bank more fully, developing and applying new assessments will become much easier. In the past, when existing tests or items became too difficult or too easy for a group of students, teachers developed separate tests for that group. That meant that scores from the newly developed tests no longer could be interpreted on the basis of the existing tests.

Using PE Metrics, teachers one day will be able to develop additional assessments targeted to the population to be tested, then link them to the existing assessment bank. That, of course, will result in the PE Metrics assessment bank growing, gradually forming a complete bank. Once that occurs, teachers will be able to propose new assessment tasks by developing the task, administering it with a PE Metrics item, and allowing PE Metrics to generate IRT statistics to equate.

Scaling & Scaled Scores

Because the difficulties of assessment tasks in the PE Metrics bank are different, teachers should not use raw scores as reflective of student ability or competence. A score of 4 from a difficult assessment simply has a different meaning than a score of 4 from an easy task. To avoid that inconsistent impact, the PE Metrics assessment bank found at www.PEMetrics.org will allow teachers to convert raw scores into an entirely different set of values called "scale scores" or "ability scores." A scale score is a transformed raw test score with different measurement units.

The scale used for the ACT college entrance test, with a mean of 22 and standard deviation (SD) of 3, provides good example of the scale scores. The ability score scale that PE Metrics employs has a mean of 500 and a SD of 100. Although teachers can still use raw scores for their informal assessment practice (formative), they should use ability scores, which PE Metrics Ability Score Calculator found at www.PEMetrics.org will calculate automatically, in all formal (summative or comparative) assessment practice.

Calibration of Standard 1 Assessments
Samples & Data Collection

This project is one of the largest and most comprehensive analyses of the current state of movement performance among middle and high school students in physical education across the country. Using the 12 middle school and eight high school Standard 1 assessments described earlier, more than 2,000 students were assessed at 45 schools. (n: middle school = 1,305, with 605 boys, 671 girls and 29 not reporting gender; n: high school = 1,046, with 559 boys, 411 girls and 76 not reporting gender.) For each class of students, at least two assessments were administered, along with at least one common assessment so that assessments within one grade can be set onto the same scale. In most cases, all assessments were given in the same week or on the same day. In addition, a selected sample was administered linking assessments so that scales across grades can be linked.

Statistical data analyses. Analyses of the national sample included extensive traditional test-construction methodology, such as item difficulty ratings and discrimination indices, which established evidence of validity. A more contemporary analysis using IRT also was applied to examine the model-data fit and to establish the item bank.

This cutting-edge approach examined item difficulty and discrimination for the purpose of equating assessments across assessments within grade levels. Equating thus allows teachers to compare students on the same scale even if different assessments are used. For example, teachers can compare middle school students using either the soccer or softball assessment. IRT-based model-data fit and categorization statistics also were established to make sure statistically that the data really represent the entire population.

Summary of Results

Tables 1-2 (pp. 27-30) summarize descriptive statistics and frequencies of assessments for middle and high school, respectively. Tables 3 and 4 (pp. 30-31) summarize the difficulty of assessments by middle and high school, respectively, according to the IRT calibrations. Note that only assessments' difficulties based on IRT were reported, and more detailed information for model-data fit statistics and corresponding information for each scoring rubric will be reported at a later date in another research publication. (For more information, visit www.aahperd.org/aapar/publications/journals.)

For an informal assessment practice, teachers can select an assessment based on its difficulty. (The larger the value, the more difficult the task; see Tables 3 and 4.) Keep in mind that the difficulty is expressed in logits, which is very much like a z-score with some negative values. Accordingly, among the middle school assessments, badminton is the most difficult, followed by pickleball and volleyball. In contrast archery is the easiest, followed by traverse climbing and softball.

After administering any assessment, teachers can compare the results with the national statistics summarized in Tables 1-2. For example, teachers who administer the high school wall climbing assessment and calculate their class average to be 2.5 on each dimension will see that the class performed slightly better than the national average. If 50 percent of the class scored a 3 on the rubric's technique dimension, the teacher can feel good about it, because nationally, only about 30 percent of high school students scored a 3 or higher.

Calibration of Standards 2-6 Assessments

Standards 2-6 assessments are cognitive test items and have been calibrated using IRT techniques, also. Following the rationale above, the cognitive items have been placed on an ability scale and can be converted to ability scores.

The content of Standard 2, which is based on exercise physiology, biomechanics, motor learning and motor development principles, stands alone. Because the contents of Standards 3 and 4 are similar, NASPE developed one bank of test items for the combined standards. Standards 5 and 6 were combined similarly.

Two forms were developed for each set of standards for both grade 8 and high school, respectively. Each form contains seven or eight common items, and through those common items, two forms are equated to the same scale. As a result, a total of 12 forms were developed. These forms were also administered to a large national sample (55 schools, 2,727 students). The sample sizes by grade, standard and form are summarized in Table 5 (p. 31).

Summary of Results

Both conventional and IRT-based item analyses were conducted for test forms for Standards 2, 3 & 4, and 5 & 6 for grade 8 and high school, respectively. Table 6 (p. 32) summarizes the criteria used for the item evaluation.

For example, Item 1 at Form A for Standard 2, grade 8 has a "good" item difficulty (0.62), as well as a "very good" and "good" discrimination based on index discrimination (0.62) and point-biserial correlation (0.54), respectively. Logit based on IRT analysis is -0.41, and both infit and outfit statistics supported a good model data fit (see Table 6). Item statistic reports for Form A by grade and standard are organized as follows:

- Table 7: Grade 8, Standard 2 (page 33).
- Table 8: Grade 8, Standards 3 & 4 (page 35).
- Table 9: Grade 8, Standards 5 & 6 (page 37).
- Table10: High School, Standard 2 (page 39).
- Table 11: High School, Standards 3 & 4 (page 41).
- Table 12: High School, Standards 5 & 6 (page 43).

Note that in each table, the item statistics for the common items are reported first, followed by the statistics for the unique items.

In contrast to Standard 1 assessments, teachers should use the entire form for the Standards 2-6 assessments when measuring a standard, although they have the option to use small numbers of questions in one standard or select small numbers of questions across all standards.

In creating these test questions, NASPE omitted any questions for which more than 90 percent of a national sample answered either correctly or incorrectly. Therefore, no question is unusually easy or difficult. The overall test difficulty was not computed, as most teachers will not administer the entire test as is.

Using PE Metrics Appropriately

Because NASPE recognizes that teachers will want to use these tests in a variety of ways, this publication offers two options:

1. This book offers printed, keyed question items from Form A related to specific standards and performance descriptors (pp. 155-186). Teachers may use these items, especially for formative assessments.

2. The CD-ROM accompanying this book also contains the test items, and teachers are encouraged to copy them into a Word document from which to administer items to students. Teachers may use entire tests for a standard or may select items across or within particular standards.

3. PE Metrics Online. Teachers from school districts that purchase NASPE's PE Metrics Online will have access to different test items, which also are linked to the same standards and performance descriptors. Teachers may select these items for tests to administer to students. In addition, PE Metrics Online users will be able to generate reports for students or parents to explain students' performance on the test.

Conclusion

Based on the analyses conducted, teachers should be confident that PE Metrics assessments provide a clear and meaningful set of attainable expectations for students. The format and descriptive information in the rubrics provide students and teachers with targets for improved performance. The cognitive items provide teachers with a basis for knowledge expected as a result of student learning. In addition, researchers benefit from data analyses that are far more thorough than traditional skills test analysis.

For a better interpretation of the meaning of the score, teachers or researchers are encouraged to use the online scoring program. As such, PE Metrics addresses the needs of teachers and students as the end users of the assessments, as well as researchers, who can use the assessments as an example of new and dynamic measurements and continue the development and analysis of future assessments that could be added to the existing test bank.

Table 1: Grade 8 Standard 1 Descriptive Statistics & Frequencies

Assessment	Mean	SD	n	% Students at Each Criterion Level				
				0	1	2	3	4
Archery								
Stance	3.22	0.89	173	0.0	2.9	22.5	24.3	50.3
Draw & Anchor	3.08	1.06	173	0.6	10.4	17.3	23.7	48.0
Release	2.95	3.02	207	0.0	15.0	19.3	21.7	44.0
Hits Target	3.02	1.22	207	1.0	18.8	10.1	16.9	53.1
Badminton								
Serve	1.92	1.007	145	0.0	48.3	17.2	28.3	06.2
Basic Strokes	1.94	1.066	145	0.0	49.7	15.9	24.8	09.7
Offensive Tactics	1.88	1.060	145	0.0	52.4	17.9	19.3	10.3
Defensive Tactics	1.83	1.063	145	0.0	57.2	11.7	22.1	09.0
Floor Hockey								
Basic Skills	2.87	0.82	86	2.3	0.0	26.7	50.0	20.9
Offensive Skills	2.48	0.98	86	3.5	10.5	34.9	37.2	14.0
Movement Without the Puck	2.83	1.03	86	3.5	7.0	20.9	40.7	27.9
Defensive Skills	3.07	1.24	86	10.5	0.0	9.3	32.6	47.7
Folk Dance								
Steps & Sequences	2.71	1.250	69	0.0	24.6	21.7	11.6	42.0
Performs to Beat of the Music	2.80	1.195	69	0.0	18.8	26.1	11.6	43.5
Synchronizes Movements With Others	3.10	0.942	69	0.0	5.8	21.7	29.0	43.5
Line Dance								
Steps & Sequences	1.76	1.024	218	0.0	59.2	13.3	19.7	7.8
Moves to the Beat of the Music	1.83	1.043	218	0.0	55.0	15.1	21.1	8.7
Pickleball								
Serve	2.17	0.916	47	0.0	27.7	34.0	31.9	6.4
Appropriate Strokes	2.70	1.214	47	0.0	25.5	14.9	23.4	36.2
Offensive Tactics	2.55	1.19	47	0.0	27.7	19.1	23.4	29.8
Defensive Tactics	2.68	1.18	47	0.0	25.5	12.8	29.8	31.9
Soccer								
Basic Skills	2.05	0.917	431	0.0	32.9	35.3	25.3	6.5
Offensive Skills	2.04	0.912	433	0.0	33.3	35.6	24.9	6.2
Movement Without the Ball	2.00	0.933	431	0.0	36.7	33.4	23.2	6.7
Defensive Skills	2.05	0.873	431	0.0	29.7	41.1	23.4	5.8

Table 1 *(Cont.)*: Grade 8 Standard 1 Descriptive Statistics & Frequencies

Assessment	Mean	SD	n	% Students at Each Criterion Level				
				0	1	2	3	4
Softball								
Fields Ground Ball	3.28	0.65	64	0.0	1.6	9.4	50.0	39.0
Transition to Throw	3.45	0.72	33	0.0	0.0	15.2	24.2	60.6
Throws to 1st Base	3.35	0.74	64	0.0	1.6	14.0	34.4	50.0
Catches a Catchable Ball at 1st Base	2.82	1.10	64	0.0	17.2	18.8	28.0	36.0
Team Handball								
Basic Skills	3.09	0.900	198	0.50	5.1	18.2	37.9	38.4
Offensive Skills	2.94	0.970	198	0.50	8.6	21.2	35.9	33.8
Movement Without the Ball	2.48	1.174	198	3.0	22.2	22.7	27.3	24.7
Defensive Tactics	2.35	1.147	198	3.0	23.7	29.3	22.7	21.2
Traverse Climbing								
Proper Technique	3.19	0.982	134	0.70	5.2	20.1	22.4	51.5
Legs for Support & Hands	2.83	1.11	134	0.0	14.2	24.6	22.4	38.1
for Balance	3.12	1.12	134	0.0	14.9	11.9	19.4	53.7
Crossover	2.68	1.330	134	0.70	31.3	10.4	14.2	43.3
Completes 20-Foot Traverse								
Ultimate Frisbee®								
Basic Skills	2.48	0.919	126	0.0	13.5	40.5	30.2	15.9
Offense	2.67	0.995	126	0.0	15.9	23.0	38.9	22.2
Defense	2.71	1.051	126	0.0	15.9	26.2	29.4	28.6
Volleyball								
Forearm Pass Criteria	1.25	1.230	235	36.2	26.0	20.9	10.6	6.4
Forearm Pass Accuracy	1.29	1.228	258	31.0	34.1	17.4	9.3	8.1
Overhead Pass Criteria	1.58	1.252	258	23.3	29.1	22.9	15.9	8.9
Overhead Pass Accuracy	1.89	1.332	258	16.7	28.3	20.9	17.8	16.3

Table 2: High School Standard 1 Descriptive Statistics & Frequencies

Assessment	Mean	SD	n	% Students at Each Criterion Level				
				0	1	2	3	4
Basketball								
Ball Skills	2.30	0.92	180	0.0	25.6	25.0	43.3	6.1
Offensive Play	2.19	0.90	180	0.0	30.0	23.9	43.3	2.8
Individual Defensive Play	2.07	0.82	180	0.0	27.2	42.2	27.2	3.3
Team Defense	2.40	0.96	180	0.0	22.2	27.2	38.9	11.7
Bowling								
Set-Up & Delivery	1.52	0.93	21	0.0	71.4	9.5	14.3	4.8
Total Bowling Score	2.14	1.28	21	0.0	42.9	28.6	0.0	28.6
Scoring	1.00	0.00	21	0.0	100.0	0.0	0.0	0.0
Flag Football								
Quarterback	2.27	0.99	94	4.3	17.0	36.2	33.0	9.6
Receiver Patterns	2.95	0.98	94	2.1	8.5	11.7	47.9	29.8
Receiver Catches	1.05	1.45	94	58.5	8.5	13.8	7.4	11.7
Defensive Player	2.41	1.06	94	6.4	16.0	16.0	53.2	8.5
Golf								
Pre-Swing	2.44	0.80	110	0.0	10.0	45.5	35.5	9.1
Full Swing	2.34	1.09	110	0.0	26.4	34.5	18.2	20.9
Ball Trajectory	1.99	1.04	70	0.0	41.4	31.4	14.3	12.9
Soccer								
Ball Control	3.16	0.79	121	0.0	1.7	19.0	41.3	38.0
Offensive Techniques	3.15	0.81	121	0.0	1.7	21.5	37.2	39.7
Defensive Techniques	3.20	0.76	121	0.0	1.7	15.7	43.8	38.8
Swimming								
Swim Prone	3.09	0.94	139	1.4	8.6	5.0	48.9	36.0
Swim Supine	2.91	0.97	139	0.0	12.9	12.2	45.3	29.5
Treads Water	3.65	0.72	139	0.0	4.1	2.0	18.4	75.5
Tennis								
Serve	1.89	1.05	37	0.0	54.1	8.1	32.4	5.4
Ground Strokes	1.46	0.77	37	0.0	70.3	13.5	16.2	0.0
Choice of Strokes	1.70	0.94	37	0.0	56.8	21.6	16.2	5.4
Hits to Open Spaces	1.46	0.84	37	0.0	73.0	10.8	13.5	2.7
Returns Ball	1.57	0.84	37	0.0	64.9	13.5	21.6	0.0
Rules	1.81	0.97	37	0.0	56.8	5.4	37.8	0.0

Table 2 *(Cont.)*: High School Standard 1 Descriptive Statistics & Frequencies

Assessment	Mean	SD	n	% Students at Each Criterion Level				
				0	**1**	**2**	**3**	**4**
Volleyball								
Forearm Passing Technique	1.61	1.18	142	26.1	14.8	34.5	21.1	3.5
Overhead Passing Technique	1.56	1.30	142	31.7	14.8	24.6	23.2	5.6
Serve	2.34	0.91	127	4.7	9.4	39.4	40.2	6.3
Wall Climbing								
Technique	2.25	0.67	85	1.2	5.9	63.5	25.9	3.5
Body Efficiency	2.24	0.84	85	1.2	16.5	45.9	30.6	5.9
Complete Climb	2.33	0.81	85	1.2	10.6	49.4	31.8	7.1
Weight Training								
Safety	3.13	0.95	537	0.6	4.7	21.8	27.0	46.0
Lifting	3.40	0.87	539	1.5	2.8	8.3	29.5	57.9
Spotting	2.22	0.79	538	2.6	3.2	75.7	7.1	11.5

Table 3: Summary of IRT Calibration of Middle School Assessments

Assessment	Difficulty Logit
Archery	-0.81
Badminton	0.71
Floor Hockey	-0.39
Folk Dance	0.18
Line Dance	0.36
Pickleball	0.67
Soccer	0.36
Softball	-0.68
Team Handball	-0.40
Traverse Climbing	-0.69
Ultimate Frisbee®	0.24
Volleyball	0.46

Table 4: Summary of IRT Calibration of High School Assessments

Assessment	Difficulty Logit
Basketball	0.30
Flag Football	-0.04
Golf	-0.04
Soccer	-0.51
Swimming	0.27
Volleyball	0.60
Wall Climbing	0.12
Weight Training	-0.70

Table 5: Sample Size Summary by Grade, Standards & Form

Grade 8	Form A	Form B
Standard 2	246	203
Standards 3 & 4	284	108
Standards 5 & 6	369	405
High School	**Form A**	**Form B**
Standard 2	159	170
Standards 3 & 4	61	326
Standards 5 & 6	208	188

Table 6: Item Analysis and Evaluation Criteria

Item Difficulty: Interpretation of Proportion Correct (Prop or P)

The proportion correct index, or, simply, "P value," is an index expressing the proportion of test takers who responded correctly to a particular item. It ranges from 0 to 1.

0 – 0.29	Too difficult
0.30 – 0.70	Good
0.71 – 0.90	Easy
0.91 – 1	Too easy

Item Discrimination: Index of Discrimination (Dis)

The range of the index of discrimination is from -1 to +1. The desirable pattern for discrimination is negative for incorrect answers and positive for the correct answers.

≥ 0.40	**Very good** (good students choose; bottom students avoid).
0.30 – 0.39	**Reasonably good** (Subject to possible improvement).
0.20 – 0.29	**Marginal items** (usually needing and subject to improvement).
< 0.20	**Poor items** (reject or improve by revision).

Item Discrimination: Point-Biserial (Point Bi or PB)

An index estimates the correlation between a single item and the total score in a test.

< 0	Very bad (delete for sure).
< 0.15	Poor
0.15 – 0.25	Marginal
> 0.25	Good

IRT Analysis

"Model Measure" explains the difficulty of an item. Negative value indicates an easier item, and positive value indicates a more difficult item. Mean difficulty is centered around zero. An item fits the Item Response Theory (Rasch) model well if its infit and outfit statistics (both in mean square residuals: MnSq) are between -2 and 2.

Table 7: Item Statistics of Common Items and Form A for Grade 8, Standard 2

Common Items

Form	Number	Prop	Dis	Point Bi	Number Correct	n	Model Measure	SE	Infit MnSq	Outfit MnSq
A/B	2	0.45	0.77	0.47	344	448	-1.15	0.12	0.9	0.9
A/B	4	0.34	0.46	0.30	207	448	0.41	0.10	1.2	1.2
A/B	5	0.35	0.60	0.34	271	448	-0.26	0.10	1.1	1.1
A/B	7	0.49	0.68	0.45	305	448	-0.65	0.11	1.0	1.0
A/B	13	0.52	0.69	0.49	309	448	-0.69	0.11	0.9	0.9
A/B	21	0.44	0.46	0.37	205	448	0.43	0.10	1.0	1.0
A/B	23	0.63	0.52	0.53	235	447	0.11	0.10	0.9	0.9
A/B	28	0.32	0.63	0.30	284	445	-0.42	0.11	1.1	1.2
A/B	32	0.29	0.42	0.29	190	444	0.57	0.10	1.2	1.2
A/B	33	0.60	0.68	0.56	306	442	-0.70	0.11	0.9	0.8
A/B	34	0.51	0.57	0.44	255	442	-0.12	0.10	0.9	0.9

Note: NA = Not available.

Form A

Form	Number	Prop	Dis	Point Bi	Number Correct	n	Model Measure	SE	Infit MnSq	Outfit MnSq
A	1	0.67	0.62	0.56	151	245	-0.43	0.14	0.9	0.8
A	3	0.42	0.55	0.38	134	245	-0.09	0.14	1.1	1.0
A	6	0.56	0.67	0.55	164	245	-0.71	0.15	0.8	0.8
A	8	0.44	0.36	0.39	87	245	0.87	0.15	1.0	1.0
A	9	0.68	0.64	0.59	156	245	-0.54	0.15	0.8	0.8
A	10	0.46	0.36	0.37	87	245	0.87	0.15	1.0	1.1
A	11	0.58	0.42	0.50	104	245	0.51	0.14	0.9	0.9
A	12	0.49	0.46	0.41	113	245	0.33	0.14	1.0	1.0
A	14	0.44	0.56	0.39	136	245	-0.13	0.14	1.1	1.1
A	15	0.65	0.47	0.53	115	245	0.29	0.14	0.9	0.9
A	16	0.59	0.53	0.49	129	244	0.00	0.14	0.9	0.9
A	17	-0.09	0.12	-0.08	30	245	2.46	0.21	1.3	2.6
A	18	0.23	0.29	0.24	70	244	1.25	0.15	1.1	1.4
A	19	0.46	0.65	0.42	160	244	-0.63	0.15	1.0	1.0
A	20	Omitted								
A	22	0.45	0.66	0.39	161	245	-0.64	0.15	1.0	1.0
A	24	0.63	0.60	0.56	147	244	-0.35	0.14	0.9	0.8
A	25	0.63	0.68	0.53	166	244	-0.76	0.15	0.8	0.8
A	26	0.51	0.60	0.44	148	243	-0.38	0.14	1.0	0.9
A	27	0.60	0.67	0.55	163	242	-0.72	0.15	0.9	0.8
A	29	0.28	0.36	0.25	88	242	0.83	0.15	1.1	1.3

Table 7 *(Cont.)*: Item Statistics of Common Items and Form A for Grade 8, Standard 2

	Conventional Analysis				Count		IRT Analysis			
Form	Number	Prop	Dis	Point Bi	Number Correct	n	Model Measure	SE	Infit MnSq	Outfit MnSq
A	30	0.49	0.72	0.48	176	242	-1.03	0.16	0.9	0.9
A	31	0.60	0.63	0.53	155	240	-0.58	0.15	0.9	0.9
A	35	0.67	0.50	0.56	123	240	0.09	0.14	0.9	0.8
A	36	0.37	0.38	0.33	92	237	0.72	0.15	1.1	1.2
A	37	0.19	0.36	0.19	88	238	0.81	0.15	1.2	1.4
A	38	0.62	0.56	0.52	137	235	-0.27	0.15	0.9	0.9
A	39	0.63	0.54	0.56	132	235	-0.16	0.14	0.9	0.8
A	40	0.04	0.23	0.05	57	231	1.49	0.17	1.3	1.9

Notes: Prop = Proportion getting right or difficulty; Dis = Index Discrimination; Point Bi = Point-Biserial;
Number Correct = Number of students getting right on this item; Model Measure = IRT item difficulty in logit;
SE = Standard Error; Infit MnSq = Infit mean square residuals; Outfit MnSq = Outfit mean square residuals.

Table 8: Item Statistics of Common Items and Form A for Grade 8, Standards 3 & 4

Common Items

	Conventional Analysis				Count		IRT Analysis			
Form	Number	Prop	Dis	Point Bi	Number Correct	n	Model Measure	SE	Infit MnSq	Outfit MnSq
A/B	3	0.74	0.46	0.47	291	391	-0.94	0.12	1.0	1.0
A/B	11	0.44	0.47	0.40	173	391	0.55	0.11	1.0	1.1
A/B	14	0.55	0.44	0.37	216	391	0.04	0.11	1.1	1.1
A/B	17	0.42	0.37	0.34	163	390	0.67	0.11	1.1	1.2
A/B	18	0.69	0.63	0.56	268	390	-0.62	0.12	0.9	0.8
A/B	21	0.57	0.61	0.49	222	390	-0.03	0.11	1.0	0.9
A/B	29	0.53	0.45	0.39	207	390	0.15	0.11	1.0	1.0
A/B	31	0.64	0.51	0.44	249	389	-0.38	0.11	1.0	1.0
A/B	36	0.57	0.46	0.43	222	389	-0.04	0.11	1.0	0.9
A/B	39	0.45	0.37	0.36	175	388	0.52	0.11	1.1	1.1

Note: NA = Not available.

Form A

	Conventional Analysis				Count		IRT Analysis			
Form	Number	Prop	Dis	Point Bi	Number Correct	n	Model Measure	SE	Infit MnSq	Outfit MnSq
A	1	0.51	0.36	0.31	145	283	0.25	0.13	1.1	1.1
A	2	0.16	0.04	0.09	46	281	2.13	0.17	1.1	1.4
A	4	0.64	0.26	0.25	181	283	-0.35	0.13	1.1	1.1
A	5	0.55	0.25	0.26	155	282	0.08	0.13	1.1	1.1
A	6	0.60	0.44	0.39	171	282	-0.19	0.13	1.0	0.9
A	7	0.83	0.39	0.51	236	283	-1.53	0.17	0.8	0.6
A	8	0.71	0.46	0.43	202	283	-0.74	0.14	1.0	0.9
A	9	0.29	0.15	0.18	81	281	1.33	0.14	1.1	1.2
A	10	0.41	0.35	0.33	116	283	0.72	0.13	1.0	1.0
A	12	0.49	0.45	0.35	140	282	0.32	0.13	1.0	1.0
A	13	0.24	0.13	0.12	67	283	1.63	0.15	1.2	1.3
A	15	0.68	0.55	0.50	192	283	-0.55	0.14	0.9	0.9
A	16	0.53	0.68	0.56	151	281	0.14	0.13	0.8	0.8
A	19	0.64	0.53	0.42	181	283	-0.35	0.13	0.9	0.9
A	20	0.37	0.17	0.15	105	283	0.91	0.13	1.2	1.3
A	22	0.64	0.46	0.37	180	283	-0.34	0.13	1.0	1.0
A	23	0.56	0.48	0.41	60	108	-0.01	0.21	1.0	1.0
A	24	0.69	0.62	0.55	194	282	-0.60	0.14	0.8	0.8
A	25	0.45	0.5	0.42	128	281	0.51	0.13	0.9	0.9
A	26	0.54	0.33	0.28	152	282	0.12	0.13	1.1	1.1

Table 8 *(Cont.)*: Item Statistics of Common Items and Form A for Grade 8, Standards 3 & 4

Conventional Analysis				Count		IRT Analysis			
Form	Number	Prop	Dis	Point Bi	Number Correct	n	Model Measure	SE	Infit MnSq	Outfit MnSq
A	27	0.60	0.54	0.47	170	283	-0.17	0.13	0.9	0.9
A	28	0.60	0.33	0.28	169	281	-0.17	0.13	1.1	1.1
A	30	0.74	0.52	0.49	209	281	-0.91	0.15	0.9	0.8
A	32	0.79	0.48	0.51	224	282	-1.24	0.16	0.8	0.7
A	33	0.49	0.41	0.31	140	281	0.32	0.13	1.1	1.1
A	34	0.46	0.49	0.40	131	281	0.47	0.13	1.0	1.0
A	35	0.73	0.43	0.42	208	281	-0.89	0.14	0.9	0.9
A	37	0.56	0.48	0.41	158	281	0.02	0.13	1.0	1.0
A	38	0.67	0.53	0.47	189	281	-0.51	0.14	0.9	0.9
A	40	0.35	0.41	0.33	100	279	0.98	0.13	1.0	1.0

Notes: Prop = Proportion getting right or difficulty; Dis = Index Discrimination; Point Bi = Point-Biserial; Number Correct = Number of students getting right on this item; Model Measure = IRT item difficulty in logit; SE = Standard Error; Infit MnSq = Infit mean square residuals; Outfit MnSq = Outfit mean square residuals.

Table 9: Item Statistics of Common Items and Form A for Grade 8, Standards 5 & 6

Common Items

| | Conventional Analysis | | | | Count | | IRT Analysis | | | |
Form	Number	Prop	Dis	Point Bi	Number Correct	n	Model Measure	SE	Infit MnSq	Outfit MnSq
A/B	2	0.93	0.20	0.49	696	752	-1.47	0.15	0.9	0.6
A/B	4	0.89	0.30	0.50	664	752	-0.84	0.13	1.0	0.8
A/B	7	0.90	0.26	0.52	678	751	-1.10	0.14	1.0	0.8
A/B	10	0.80	0.45	0.55	600	752	0.02	0.11	1.0	0.9
A/B	11	0.85	0.40	0.64	636	751	-0.43	0.12	0.8	0.6
A/B	14	0.41	0.47	0.37	298	750	2.41	0.08	1.2	1.3
A/B	15	0.71	0.59	0.56	527	751	0.72	0.09	1.0	1.0
A/B	16	0.77	0.55	0.62	574	752	0.29	0.10	0.9	0.8
A/B	19	0.85	0.42	0.60	634	750	-0.41	0.12	0.9	0.7
A/B	22	0.85	0.39	0.61	639	752	-0.46	0.12	0.9	0.9
A/B	25	0.91	0.27	0.60	679	750	-1.14	0.14	0.8	0.6
A/B	28	0.55	0.60	0.42	408	751	1.63	0.08	1.1	1.2
A/B	31	0.85	0.42	0.62	633	751	-0.39	0.12	0.8	0.6
A/B	38	0.77	0.47	0.54	572	749	0.30	0.10	1.0	1.0
A/B	40	0.82	0.42	0.56	610	741	-0.19	0.11	0.9	0.8

Note: NA = Not available.

Form A

| | Conventional Analysis | | | | Count | | IRT Analysis | | | |
Form	Number	Prop	Dis	Point Bi	Number Correct	n	Model Measure	SE	Infit MnSq	Outfit MnSq
A	1	0.85	0.30	0.28	300	355	-0.10	0.17	1.3	1.1
A	3	0.90	0.14	0.24	320	355	-0.75	0.20	1.2	1.4
A	5	0.86	0.25	0.37	303	355	-0.19	0.17	1.1	1.2
A	6	0.95	0.12	0.45	337	355	-1.60	0.26	0.9	0.6
A	8	0.79	0.30	0.38	279	355	0.41	0.15	1.2	1.4
A	9	0.85	0.32	0.42	298	355	-0.05	0.16	1.1	0.9
A	12	0.69	0.43	0.45	241	355	1.13	0.13	1.0	1.0
A	13	0.93	0.19	0.58	328	355	-1.10	0.22	0.8	0.6
A	17	0.86	0.33	0.54	302	355	-0.16	0.17	0.9	0.7
A	18	0.88	0.30	0.53	310	354	-0.43	0.18	0.9	0.6
A	20	0.85	0.40	0.65	298	353	-0.07	0.17	0.8	0.6
A	21	0.86	0.37	0.64	304	355	-0.21	0.17	0.8	0.6
A	23	0.82	0.28	0.40	287	355	0.23	0.15	1.1	1.3
A	24	0.85	0.30	0.53	299	355	-0.07	0.17	0.9	1.0
A	26	0.80	0.43	0.49	283	355	0.32	0.15	1.0	0.9
A	27	0.84	0.36	0.62	296	355	0.01	0.16	0.8	0.8
A	29	0.68	0.35	0.36	239	354	1.15	0.13	1.2	1.2
A	30	0.66	0.44	0.35	230	354	1.30	0.13	1.2	1.3

Table 9 *(Cont.)*: Item Statistics of Common Items and Form A for Grade 8, Standards 5 & 6

Conventional Analysis				Count		IRT Analysis			
Form	Number	Prop	Dis	Point Bi	Number Correct	n	Model Measure	SE	Infit MnSq	Outfit MnSq
A	32	0.85	0.42	0.70	300	354	-0.13	0.17	0.7	0.4
A	33	0.75	0.41	0.50	264	354	0.70	0.14	1.0	1.0
A	34	0.74	0.49	0.56	258	354	0.81	0.14	0.9	0.9
A	35	0.64	0.37	0.34	224	354	1.39	0.13	1.2	1.4
A	36	0.90	0.24	0.56	317	354	-0.67	0.19	0.9	0.7
A	37	0.83	0.31	0.50	291	352	0.09	0.16	1.0	1.1
A	39	0.84	0.33	0.46	297	352	-0.08	0.17	1.0	0.8

Notes: Prop = Proportion getting right or difficulty; Dis = Index Discrimination; Point Bi = Point-Biserial;

Number Correct = Number of students getting right on this item; Model Measure = IRT item difficulty in logit;

SE = Standard Error; Infit MnSq = Infit mean square residuals; Outfit MnSq = Outfit mean square residuals.

Table 10: Item Statistics of Common Items and Form A for High School, Standard 2

Common Items

		Conventional Analysis			Count		IRT Analysis			
Form	Number	Prop	Dis	Point Bi	Number Correct	n	Model Measure	SE	Infit MnSq	Outfit MnSq
A/B	1	0.39	0.16	0.12	128	330	0.37	0.12	1.1	1.2
A/B	2	0.57	0.28	0.24	187	329	-0.45	0.12	1.0	1.1
A/B	7	0.31	0.18	0.20	101	329	0.77	0.13	1.0	1.1
A/B	9	0.44	0.51	0.43	144	329	0.15	0.12	0.9	0.9
A/B	10	0.71	0.10	0.15	234	330	-1.13	0.13	1.1	1.1
A/B	18	0.59	0.46	0.38	193	329	-0.53	0.12	1.0	1.0
A/B	25	0.72	0.63	0.54	238	327	-1.23	0.13	0.8	0.7
A/B	38	0.39	0.42	0.38	128	326	0.35	0.12	1.0	1.0
A/B	39	0.26	-0.01	-0.01	87	326	0.98	0.13	1.2	1.3

Note: NA = Not available.

Form A

		Conventional Analysis			Count		IRT Analysis			
Form	Number	Prop	Dis	Point Bi	Number Correct	n	Model Measure	SE	Infit MnSq	Outfit MnSq
A	3	0.35	0.13	0.15	111	156	-0.96	0.19	0.9	0.9
A	4	0.56	0.18	0.12	110	157	-0.91	0.18	1.1	1.1
A	6	0.54	0.53	0.42	100	157	-0.59	0.18	1.1	1.1
A	8	0.62	0.17	0.19	49	157	0.92	0.18	1.2	1.3
A	11	0.77	0.42	0.39	142	157	-2.41	0.28	1.0	0.8
A	12	0.83	0.47	0.53	71	157	0.25	0.17	1.0	1.0
A	13	0.52	0.55	0.45	81	156	-0.04	0.17	1.0	1.0
A	14	0.22	-0.06	-0.06	106	156	-0.79	0.18	0.9	0.8
A	15	0.70	0.53	0.46	57	157	0.67	0.17	1.2	1.2
A	16	0.70	0.26	0.25	78	157	0.05	0.17	1.0	0.9
A	20	0.31	-0.04	0.03	67	157	0.37	0.17	1.1	1.1
A	21	0.90	0.21	0.32	40	157	1.23	0.19	1.1	1.2
A	22	0.45	0.30	0.29	69	156	0.3	0.17	1.1	1.1
A	23	0.51	0.37	0.33	87	157	-0.2	0.17	1.0	1.0
A	24	0.67	0.62	0.51	72	157	0.23	0.17	0.9	0.9
A	26	0.36	0.03	0.07	114	157	-1.05	0.19	0.8	0.7
A	27	0.49	0.46	0.40	108	157	-0.84	0.18	0.9	0.9
A	28	0.09	0.01	0.03	107	157	-0.81	0.18	0.9	0.8
A	29	0.17	0.10	0.10	90	157	-0.29	0.17	0.9	0.9
A	30	0.42	0.25	0.21	126	157	-1.51	0.21	0.8	0.6
A	31	0.25	0.12	0.16	116	157	-1.12	0.19	0.9	0.9

Table 10 *(Cont.)*: Item Statistics of Common Items and Form A for High School, Standard 2

Conventional Analysis				Count		IRT Analysis			
Form	Number	Prop	Dis	Point Bi	Number Correct	n	Model Measure	SE	Infit MnSq	Outfit MnSq
A	32	0.44	0.24	0.23	110	155	-0.95	0.19	1.0	1.1
A	33	0.55	0.49	0.35	71	155	0.24	0.17	0.9	0.9
A	34	0.46	0.47	0.41	89	155	-0.29	0.17	1.1	1.1
A	35	0.72	0.70	0.63	75	155	0.12	0.17	1.0	0.9
A	36	0.68	0.52	0.48	82	155	-0.08	0.17	0.9	0.9
A	37	0.68	0.60	0.51	78	154	0.03	0.17	0.9	0.9
A	40	0.57	0.57	0.47	36	155	1.37	0.20	1.1	1.1

Notes: Prop = Proportion getting right or difficulty; Dis = Index Discrimination; Point Bi = Point-Biserial;

Number Correct = Number of students getting right on this item; Model Measure = IRT item difficulty in logit;

SE = Standard Error; Infit MnSq = Infit mean square residuals; Outfit MnSq = Outfit mean square residuals.

Table 11: Item Statistics of Common Items and Form A for High School, Standards 3 & 4

Common Items

	Conventional Analysis				Count		IRT Analysis			
Form	Number	Prop	Dis	Point Bi	Number Correct	n	Model Measure	SE	Infit MnSq	Outfit MnSq
A/B	1	0.51	0.59	0.49	198	386	0.60	0.11	1.1	1.1
A/B	2	0.54	0.59	0.50	210	382	0.43	0.12	1.1	1.1
A/B	7	0.30	0.27	0.30	114	386	1.74	0.12	1.2	1.6
A/B	9	0.58	0.68	0.59	222	382	0.26	0.12	0.9	-0.9
A/B	10	0.76	0.46	0.53	295	385	-0.81	0.13	0.9	1.0
A/B	18	0.82	0.41	0.58	318	385	-1.27	0.15	0.8	-0.6
A/B	25	0.40	0.50	0.45	154	385	1.18	0.12	1.1	1.2
A/B	38	0.53	0.62	0.55	205	375	0.43	0.12	1.0	-0.9
A/B	39	0.75	0.40	0.45	288	376	-0.82	0.14	1.0	1.0

Note: NA = Not available.

Form A

	Conventional Analysis				Count		IRT Analysis			
Form	Number	Prop	Dis	Point Bi	Number Correct	n	Model Measure	SE	Infit MnSq	Outfit MnSq
A	10	0.50	0.24	0.23	30	60	0.64	0.28	1.1	1.2
A	11	0.88	0.19	0.30	53	60	-1.68	0.42	1.0	0.9
A	12	0.30	0.01	0.05	18	60	1.62	0.30	1.2	1.6
A	13	0.55	0.41	0.37	33	60	0.41	0.28	1.0	1.0
A	14	0.65	0.44	0.37	39	60	-0.08	0.29	1.0	0.9
A	15	0.67	0.58	0.42	40	60	-0.17	0.30	1.0	1.0
A	16	0.75	0.51	0.54	45	60	-0.64	0.32	0.8	-0.7
A	17	0.80	0.63	0.62	48	60	-0.97	0.34	0.8	-0.6
A	18	0.53	0.58	0.43	32	60	0.48	0.28	1.0	1.0
A	19	0.83	0.39	0.52	50	60	-1.22	0.37	0.8	0.8
A	20	0.78	0.44	0.47	47	60	-0.85	0.34	0.9	0.8
A	21	0.67	0.63	0.56	40	60	-0.17	0.30	0.8	-0.8
A	22	0.47	0.48	0.33	28	60	0.80	0.28	1.1	1.1
A	23	0.78	0.45	0.53	47	60	-0.85	0.34	0.8	-0.7
A	24	0.60	0.28	0.26	36	60	0.17	0.29	1.1	1.1
A	25	0.75	0.33	0.39	45	60	-0.64	0.32	1.0	1.0
A	26	0.48	0.29	0.26	29	60	0.72	0.28	1.1	1.2
A	27	0.55	0.30	0.32	33	60	0.41	0.28	1.0	1.1
A	28	0.87	0.38	0.44	52	60	-1.51	0.4	0.9	0.8
A	29	0.73	0.63	0.49	44	60	-0.54	0.31	0.9	-0.8
A	30	0.25	0.15	0.20	15	60	1.90	0.32	1.2	1.2
A	31	0.35	0.42	0.25	21	60	1.36	0.29	1.1	1.1

Table 11 *(Cont.)*: Item Statistics of Common Items and Form A for High School, Standards 3 & 4

	Conventional Analysis				Count		IRT Analysis			
Form	Number	Prop	Dis	Point Bi	Number Correct	n	Model Measure	SE	Infit MnSq	Outfit MnSq
A	32	0.53	0.58	0.42	32	60	0.48	0.28	1.0	1.0
A	33	0.43	0.37	0.33	26	60	0.95	0.28	1.1	1.1
A	34	0.75	0.45	0.43	45	60	-0.64	0.32	0.9	1.0
A	35	0.58	0.52	0.41	35	60	0.25	0.28	1.0	1.0
A	36	0.75	0.50	0.46	45	60	-0.64	0.32	0.9	0.8
A	37	0.62	0.58	0.49	37	58	-0.01	0.3	0.9	0.9
A	38	0.32	0.54	0.46	19	59	1.51	0.3	0.9	0.9
A	39	0.77	0.39	0.27	46	59	-0.83	0.34	1.1	1.2

Notes: Prop = Proportion getting right or difficulty; Dis = Index Discrimination; Point Bi = Point-Biserial; Number Correct = Number of students getting right on this item; Model Measure = IRT item difficulty in logit; SE = Standard Error; Infit MnSq = Infit mean square residuals; Outfit MnSq = Outfit mean square residuals.

Table 12: Item Statistics of Common Items and Form A for High School, Standards 5 & 6

Common Items

| Form | Number | Conventional Analysis | | | Count | | IRT Analysis | | | |
		Prop	Dis	Point Bi	Number Correct	n	Model Measure	SE	Infit MnSq	Outfit MnSq
A/B	8	0.82	0.39	0.50	322	391	-0.73	0.15	1.0	0.9
A/B	9	0.81	0.43	0.54	318	392	-0.63	0.15	0.9	0.9
A/B	10	0.68	0.61	0.52	265	392	0.34	0.13	1.0	1.0
A/B	12	0.83	0.51	0.69	324	391	-0.77	0.15	0.7	0.5
A/B	14	0.81	0.52	0.65	315	391	-0.57	0.15	0.8	0.6
A/B	15	0.84	0.43	0.62	330	391	-0.91	0.16	0.8	0.5
B	16	0.61	0.60	0.48	237	390	0.75	0.12	1.1	1.1
A	20	0.70	0.70	0.65	272	391	0.22	0.13	0.8	0.7
A/B	21	0.77	0.52	0.56	301	390	-0.30	0.14	1.0	1.1
A/B	26	0.84	0.53	0.73	301	390	-0.30	0.14	0.9	0.9
A/B	28	0.71	0.63	0.58	330	391	-0.91	0.16	0.7	0.4
A/B	29	0.56	0.55	0.43	276	391	0.16	0.13	1.0	0.9
A/B	30	0.65	0.69	0.58	217	389	1.03	0.12	1.2	1.4
A/B	32	0.76	0.61	0.59	252	390	0.53	0.12	1.0	1.0
A/B	33	0.69	0.66	0.54	295	389	-0.19	0.14	0.9	0.8
A/B	34	0.72	0.64	0.59	268	388	0.27	0.13	1.0	0.9
A/B	36	0.84	0.27	0.43	281	388	0.04	0.13	0.9	0.9

Note: NA = Not available.

Form A

| Form | Number | Conventional Analysis | | | Count | | IRT Analysis | | | |
		Prop	Dis	Point Bi	Number Correct	n	Model Measure	SE	Infit MnSq	Outfit MnSq
A	1	0.56	0.47	0.38	115	207	1.27	0.16	1.1	1.1
A	2	0.33	0.21	0.16	69	207	2.43	0.16	1.3	1.7
A	3	0.96	0.11	0.45	199	207	-2.31	0.38	0.8	0.4
A	4	0.83	0.44	0.55	170	207	-0.37	0.20	0.9	0.7
A	5	0.75	0.36	0.39	155	207	0.17	0.18	1.1	1.1
A	6	Omitted								
A	7	0.92	0.17	0.33	191	207	-1.50	0.28	1.0	1.0
A	11	0.81	0.39	0.47	167	207	-0.25	0.20	1.0	0.9
A	13	0.66	0.50	0.45	136	207	0.73	0.17	1.0	1.0
A	17	Omitted								
A	18	0.71	0.36	0.37	147	207	0.42	0.17	1.1	1.2
A	19	0.80	0.45	0.58	166	207	-0.21	0.19	0.9	0.8
A	20	0.70	0.70	0.65	272	391	0.22	0.13	0.8	0.7

Table 12 *(Cont.)*: Item Statistics of Common Items and Form A for High School, Standards 5 & 6

	Conventional Analysis				Count		IRT Analysis			
Form	Number	Prop	Dis	Point Bi	Number Correct	n	Model Measure	SE	Infit MnSq	Outfit MnSq
A	22	0.58	0.55	0.39	120	207	1.15	0.16	1.1	1.2
A	23	0.88	0.34	0.54	183	207	-0.98	0.24	0.8	0.5
A	24	0.78	0.34	0.40	162	207	-0.06	0.19	1.1	1.2
A	25	0.82	0.39	0.50	170	207	-0.37	0.20	0.9	0.8
A	27	0.88	0.34	0.58	183	207	-0.98	0.24	0.8	0.5
A	31	0.77	0.45	0.52	159	207	0.04	0.18	0.9	0.8
A	35	0.51	0.49	0.32	105	207	1.52	0.16	1.1	1.3
A	37	0.79	0.45	0.48	163	206	-0.13	0.19	1.0	0.9
A	38	0.83	0.45	0.61	172	206	-0.49	0.21	0.8	0.7
A	39	0.70	0.53	0.54	144	206	0.48	0.17	1.0	0.9
A	40	Omitted								

Notes: Prop = Proportion getting right or difficulty; Dis = Index Discrimination; Point Bi = Point-Biserial; Number Correct = Number of students getting right on this item; Model Measure = IRT item difficulty in logit; SE = Standard Error; Infit MnSq = Infit mean square residuals; Outfit MnSq = Outfit mean square residuals.

Chapter 5

Frequently Asked Questions About PE Metrics

Over the years of developing PE Metrics, teachers have asked many questions at conference presentations and during conversations. In this chapter, we have summarized the most frequently asked questions, and present our responses.

Q: It's so overwhelming to think about all this assessment. How can I get started?

A: Begin with small, manageable steps, such as starting your assessments with a favorite unit. You can learn how to administer an assessment with those skills that you're very confident teaching and evaluating, and introduce procedures and responsibilities to the students gradually. If problems arise, you can make changes for the next time.

You also can conduct PE Metrics assessments for a few activities in each grade level per year. For example, you might wish to assess only your eighth-graders to see how well they meet the criteria in the team sports or dance that you've focused on.

Some other ideas:

- Share or develop new assessments with your teaching colleagues before assessing students. More perspectives will help you avoid ineffective assessments and save revision time later.

- Practice and score the assessment with a few students.

- Give and score the assessment with one class of students before using the data to make instruction decisions.

- Choose a limited number of Standards 2-6 questions that might fit your curriculum and then use them as examples to develop your own questions.

Challenge yourself to work with your colleagues in your district and try conducting a sequence of assessments of similar tasks from middle to high school. For example, use the volleyball assessments for grade 8 and high school, or use the sequence of grade 8 traverse climb and high school wall climbing if you teach adventure activities. *Remember:* Developing your assessment system is a process that takes time and effort, and trial and error. You and your students need to learn the assessments first before you can collect consistent information to contribute to student learning.

Q: I don't teach many of the activities in the PE Metrics Standard 1 assessments. How can they help me?

A: PE Metrics is designed to reflect a consensus of critical outcomes and provide examples of assessments. We encourage you to use the assessments in PE Metrics as a foundation for developing your own assessments that align with your teaching objectives. Consider the Standard 1 rubrics to be templates. For example, you could modify the soccer or team handball rubric to assess floor hockey or any other invasion game, because many of the essential criteria are similar. Or look at the racket sports assessments for ideas for creating your own assessments for other racket sports.

If you develop your own assessments, remember that each criterion in the Standard 1 assessments should include only essential elements. Including too many elements in one criterion makes understanding and scoring difficult.

Q: In regard to the Standards 2-6 tests, what if I don't teach everything in the test bank?

A: You should choose those questions from the bank that fit your curriculum. In other words, if you teach fitness concepts at all grade levels, choose questions that assess those concepts specifically. You also could modify your curriculum to address more concepts in Standards 2-6.

Q: What if I want to assess my students at levels other than the end of grade 8 or high school?

A: The assessments in PE Metrics are designed as exit criteria for each standard at the designated grade level: grade 8 and high school. However, you can use any of the assessments for other grade levels, as appropriate. For example, if your high school students take physical education only in grade 9 or have physical education only one day a week, the grade 8 assessments might be more appropriate for your situation.

Also, if you have a high school student with disabilities and he or she demonstrates the gross motor or cognitive development of a younger child, it might be more appropriate to assess that student using a grade 8 or even a grade 5 assessment from the elementary assessment book, *PE Metrics: Assessing National Standards 1-6 in Elementary School.*

Conversely, if some grade 6 or 7 students have achieved Level 3 competence in a grade 8 assessment, you might challenge them by introducing them to the higher-level skills identified in the high school assessments.

Q: I have collected a lot of assessment scores from my students. What can I do with the data?

A: Here are some suggestions:

- Use the scores to demonstrate student improvement over time.
- Use the evidence of student learning to advocate for your program at the school and district levels.
- Provide summary reports for parents on their students' progress.
- Use the scores to identify strengths and weakness in your program and then, to plan your curriculum.
- Provide feedback to students on their level of performance.
- Write a brief article on your students' accomplishments for a school or district newsletter.
- Use the assessment data as feedback on your teaching. Are your students learning what you think you're teaching them?
- Add to the PE Metrics National Database in PE Metrics Online.

Q: How can I use the results of the PE Metrics assessments to assign a grade?

A: While it might be tempting to convert the rubric scores (0-4) to letter grades (A, B, C, etc.), the raw scores from the PE Metrics assessments should not be used as a grade. Rubric scores from one assessment are not necessary equal to those from another assessment. For example, a rubric score of 3 in volleyball is not equal to a score of 3 in the soccer assessment, because the tasks are not equal in difficulty.

To compare scores from one assessment to another, you must convert them to ability scores. Ability scores range from 200 to 800 and allow comparisons between various assessments, such as soccer and volleyball for grade 8. A 500 score is an indicator of competence. It's analogous to being in the Healthy Fitness Zone (HFZ). A score of 600 might indicate more fluid movement or more ability, but certainly not perfection. It's the same as being at the top of the HFZ: more is not better; both are fit. In this case, any ability score above 500 means that the student is skilled.

You can determine the ability score for a specific test by accessing PE Metrics Online. For more details, see the section on grading in Using PE Metrics Assessments.

Q: I don't have the exact equipment — such as a team handball — or space that the assessments call for. Can I substitute another ball or reduce the size of the space?

A: Yes, you can, if you're using the assessment for your own students only. You can adjust the equipment, space or trials to meet your needs, so long as you make the same changes for all students. If, however, you change the assessment again in the following semester or year, you can't compare your own classes over time or your classes with someone else's classes. You must be consistent if you want to compare student scores over time. Note that substituting equipment or space alters the assessment significantly. The assessment won't be the same without following the procedures and equipment requirements exactly as written. While physical education teachers are used to "making do," if you change any aspect of the assessments in PE Metrics, you can't compare your students' scores to the national scores or upload scores into the national PE Metrics database.

Q: PE Metrics recommends video-recording the assessments for Standard 1. Why should I video-record the assessments?

A: Problems in performance are easy to miss when you're involved in teaching. Video-recording allows you to go back and review a student's performance. Also, if you're assessing for summative assessment, you will find it helpful to have a video record of student performance, because you then will have solid evidence for documenting student achievement.

Q: I don't have time to video my classes and then view the recordings. Can I just score students "live" as they complete the assessments in class?

A: You can do that for some assessments but you will be more consistent and accurate if you record student performance and view it later. If the skill is less complicated (e.g., softball fielding or catching), you can score "live" on the score sheet or personal digital assistant. We recommend recording more complex assessments, particularly team sports, so that you can view each student individually and more than once, if necessary. The more you do that, the easier it gets and the more efficient you become. You also will find that your analysis of students' performance will be improved.

Q: What are the procedures used in Standard 1 outlined in the chapter titled Administering & Scoring PE Metrics Assessments, and why are they important?

A: The procedures in each assessment provide information on exactly how to administer the assessments. Following the procedures exactly as written provides valid and reliable skills assessment and allows for comparisons to students across the country through the PE Metrics National Database.

Q: How can I supervise my class, operate the video camera and ensure meaningful participation in my large classes and still conduct Standard 1 assessments?

A: It's challenging to maintain control of the class and ensure that all students are participating safely in an activity while you're conducting the assessments. Here are some suggestions:

- Assess in groups, if possible. Many of the assessments suggest having more than one student perform at one time. If you're video-recording for later viewing, students might be able to perform in larger groups.

- Use a number of stations related to the class objective, in which students work in small groups rotating from station to station, one of which can be the assessment station. For example, you can assess students at one station, making sure that you can see the entire teaching space while you're assessing. Other groups of students could be peer-assessing, practicing the actual assessment or self-assessing. Or, they could be working on other skills related to your current or past activities. You need to have taught students how to work in groups at stations and have clear directions for the task at each station.

- You don't need to assess all of your students on the same day; take 10 minutes out of selected class periods and assess a handful of students.

- If you have a college intern or observer, use him or her for supervision or video-recording.

- At the middle and high school levels, you and your colleagues are going to have to help each other carry out meaningful assessments for your students.

Q: I have my students only twice a week for one year. How can I use PE Metrics assessments without taking up half of my teaching time?

A: Here are some suggestions:

- You don't need to assess everyone on the same day. Take 10 or 15 minutes out of a class and assess a handful of students. The assessments can be completed over several days.

- Ask for help from older students, parents, coaches or community volunteers.

- Assess in groups, if possible, to save time.

- If the assessment is more game-like and complicated, try breaking it into parts and assess one criterion of the assessment at one time. For example, in the high school basketball assessment, you might be able to watch while students are participating in 3-v-3 game play and observe the ball-skills aspect of the assessment.

We strongly believe that the use of assessments represents a learning opportunity for students, not lost teaching time. Instruction that includes assessment provides important feedback to students regarding achievement. In other words, assessment should be part of instruction, and students should be learning how well they're meeting the criteria when participating in the assessment.

Q: How am I to use the PE Metrics Web site?

A: The PE Metrics site, www.PEMetrics.org, is designed to help you use the observation rubrics accurately. The site provides a video example of competent performance and common errors for each of the Standard 1 assessments. Before you score students on an assessment, it will help to access the video for that assessment and review the expectations for performing each level of the rubric.

Q: What is the PE Metrics National Database and why should I consider contributing to it?

A: NASPE is in the process of creating PE Metrics Online, a Web site that will allow teachers who administer the tests using the correct protocols to add their scores to the national database. If you choose to upload your students' scores, they will be added to all the other national data. In that way, the database can be updated with scores from across the country, and you can contribute to our profession's leading efforts in assessment.

Standard 1 Assessments

Grade 8 Assessments
Archery
Badminton
Floor Hockey
Folk Dance
Line Dance
Pickleball
Soccer
Softball
Team Handball
Transverse Climbing
Ultimate Frisbee®
Volleyball

High School Assessments
Basketball
Bowling
Canoeing
Flag Football
Golf
Soccer
Swimming
Tennis
Volleyball
Wall Climbing
Weight Training

Standard 1:

Demonstrates competency in motor skills and movement patterns needed to perform a variety of physical activities.

Performance Indicator:

Perform the skills and tactics of individual competitive sports in a game-like situation.

Assessment Task:

Shoot arrows into the target from 10 yards.

Criteria for Competence (Level 3):

1. Uses a stance partially parallel to the shooting line (front foot pointing toward target, back foot parallel), with shoulder of bow arm toward the target.
2. Uses a full draw and anchor position on at least 4 of 6 attempts.
3. Uses a smooth release on at least 4 of 6 attempts.
4. Hits the target face with at least 3 of 6 arrows.

■ Assessment Rubric:

Level	1. Stance	2. Draw & Anchor	3. Release	4. Hits Target
4	Consistently uses a stance with feet parallel to the shooting line and shoulder of the bow arm toward the target.	Uses a full draw and anchor position on at least 5 of 6 attempts.	Uses a smooth release on at least 5 of 6 attempts.	Hits the target face with at least 4 of 6 arrows.
3	Usually uses a stance parallel to the shooting line, with shoulder of the bow arm toward the target.	Uses a full draw and anchor position on at least 4 of 6 attempts.	Uses a smooth release on at least 4 of 6 attempts.	Hits the target face with at least 3 of 6 arrows.
2	Uses a stance with front foot toward target and shoulder open.	Uses a full draw and anchor position on 3 of 6 attempts.	Uses a smooth release on 3 of 6 attempts.	Hits the target face with 2 of 6 arrows.
1	Uses a stance with both feet and shoulders facing the target.	Uses a full draw and anchor position on fewer than 3 attempts.	Uses a smooth release on fewer than 3 of 6 attempts.	Hits the target face with 1 or fewer arrows.
0	Violates safety procedures and/or does not complete the assessment task.			

*For Level 3, students may have front foot facing partially forward.

Scoring: Consistently = 90% or above; Usually = 75% – 89%; Sometimes = 50% – 74%; Seldom = below 50%

■ Assessment Protocols:

Directions for Students (Read aloud, verbatim):

- You will shoot 1 end of 6 arrows at a target 10 yards from the shooting line.

- You will be assessed on your ability to:
    a) Use a stance parallel to the shooting line, with shoulder of the bow arm toward target.
    b) Use a full draw and anchor position.
    c) Use a smooth release.
    d) Hit the target face.

- All safety rules must be followed, including proper nocking of the arrow.

Directions for Teachers:

Preparation:

- See the chapter titled Administering & Scoring PE Metrics Assessments for instruction and warm-up.

- Establish safety and shooting procedures, and related signals.

- Have the rest of the class practice while you are filming the student being assessed.

- Move the camera only once, and only to film the students who draw the bow with the opposite (left) arm. Move to the opposite end of the shooting line.

- Because it is difficult to see whether or not an arrow hits the target on the video, score the "hits target" portion of the assessment immediately after the assessment task for each student.

Safety:

- Insist that students follow all safety rules:
    - Bow and arrow selection.
    - Well-maintained equipment.
    - Wait for signal to shoot.
    - Front foot at shooting line.
    - Nock arrow on signal.
    - Aim only at ground or target.
    - Stop on signal.
    - Cross shooting line only on signal to retrieve arrows.

- Check arrows and bows for proper maintenance, size and weight.

- Set up targets with a backdrop to stop wayward arrows or with sufficient clear space beyond the targets.

- Areas around and behind the targets must be marked to prevent anyone from entering the line of fire.

- All students must wear protective gear (arm guards, finger tabs) and proper clothing. Permit no jewelry and no objects in shirt pockets.

- All students must adhere to shooting, retrieval and emergency signals.

Equipment/Materials:

- 2 targets for assessment for 4 students; additional targets for other students.

- 2 target stands for assessment; additional target stands for other students.

- Properly sized bows and arrows for each student, ground quivers, arm guard and finger tab for each student.

- Safety net or other backdrop to collect stray arrows (if indoors).

- Numbered pinnies on front <u>and</u> back.

Diagram of Space/Distances:

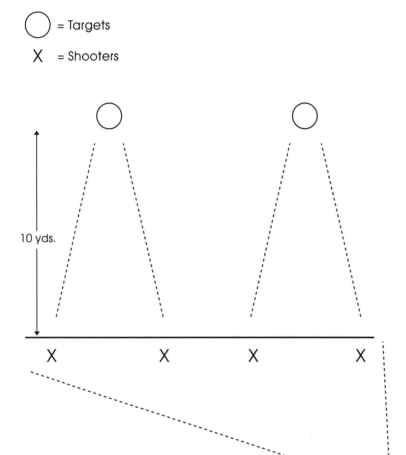

Camera Location/Operation

Set up video camera on a tripod so that the camera does not need to be moved during the shooting. Camera should be located to the bow side (right) and behind the shooters (reverse for left handed shooters) so that range of view includes the shooters and the target. The shooting line for 4 shooters should be visible. The feet of each shooter must be visible.

Assessment Score Sheet

PE Teacher _____   Grade _____   Date _____

School _____   Class Period _____

Pinnie Number	Student Name	Gender	Stance (0-4)	Draw & Anchor (0-4)	Release (0-4)	Hits Target (0-4)	Total Score (0-16) 12=Competent

Standard 1:

Demonstrates competency in motor skills and movement patterns needed to perform a variety of physical activities.

Performance Indicator:

Perform the skills and tactics of dual competitive sports in a game-like situation.

Assessment Task:

Play a competitive game of singles badminton.

Criteria for Competence (Level 3):

1. Uses a legal serve to place the shuttlecock into opponent's service area at least 8 out of 10 serves.

2. Usually chooses appropriate strokes (e.g., forehand, backhand, underhand).

3. Usually uses an offensive shot to hit the shuttle away from opponent to open space or uses a hard drive or smash to the opponent.

4. Usually moves to home base and ready position following strokes.

■ **Assessment Rubric:**

Level	1. Serve	2. Basic Strokes	3. Offensive Tactics	4. Defensive Tactics
4	Uses a legal serve to place the shuttlecock into opponent's service area 10 out of 10 serves.	Consistently chooses appropriate strokes.	Consistently uses an offensive shot to hit the shuttle away from opponent to open space or uses a hard drive or smash to the opponent.	Consistently moves to home base and ready position following strokes.
3	Uses a legal serve to place the shuttlecock into opponent's service area at least 8 out of 10 serves.	Usually chooses appropriate strokes.	Usually uses an offensive shot to hit the shuttle away from opponent to open space or uses a hard drive or smash to the opponent.	Usually moves to home base and ready position following strokes.
2	Uses a legal serve to place the shuttlecock into opponent's service area at least 6 out of 10 serves.	Sometimes chooses appropriate strokes.	Sometimes uses an offensive shot to hit the shuttle away from opponent to open space or uses a hard drive or smash to the opponent.	Sometimes moves to home base and ready position following strokes.
1	Uses a legal serve to place the shuttlecock into opponent's service area on 5 or fewer serves.	Seldom chooses appropriate strokes.	Seldom uses an offensive shot to hit the shuttle away from opponent to open space or uses a hard drive or smash to the opponent.	Seldom moves to home base and ready position following strokes.
0	Violates safety procedures and/or does not complete the assessment task.			

Scoring: Consistently = 90% or above; Usually = 75% – 89%; Sometimes = 50% –74%; Seldom = below 50%

■ **Assessment Protocols:**

Directions for Students (Read aloud, verbatim):

- You will play singles badminton.

- You will be assessed on your ability to:
    a) Use a legal serve to place the shuttlecock into your opponent's service area.
    b) Select overhand, backhand or underhand strokes appropriately.
    c) Use an offensive shot to hit the shuttle away from opponent to open space or use a hard drive or smash to the oponent.
    d) Move to home base and ready position following all strokes.

- Start play: Play will begin with the service by the player on the side opposite the camera, who will serve 10 times.

- Play on each serve will continue until the point is won/lost. No score is to be recorded.

- Alternate service to the right and left service area. Call line violations on your side of the court.

- Change side and server at completion of 10 serves.

Directions for Teachers:

Preparation:

- See the chapter titled Administering & Scoring PE Metrics Assessments for instruction and warm-up.

- Select players of similar ability as opponents.

- No score is to be kept.

- So that skills can be viewed from the same angle for both players, play should continue until one player completes 10 serves (with play after each serve continuing until the point is ended). Change sides at the completion of 10 serves.

- All rules (with the exception of scoring and change of service) should apply.

- Players will call line violations on their respective sides of the court.

Safety:

- Courts are to be dry and clear of obstruction, with adequate out-of-bounds space surrounding all sides.

- Rackets should be inspected for loose heads, handles and/or shafts.

- Other students should not be permitted to walk behind court during play.

Equipment/Materials:

- Nets, standards, and floor markings for each court.

- Racket for each player and at least 2 shuttles for each court.

- Numbered pinnies.

Diagram of Space/Distances:

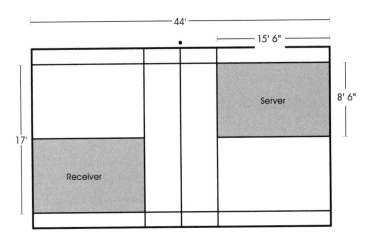

Regulation Badminton Court
Use Singles Markings

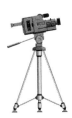

Camera Location and Operation:

Place the camera at corner of court, so that both end lines and side lines are visible at edges of the viewing screen. Place camera so that all play is in view without moving/panning during play.

Assessment Score Sheet

PE Teacher ....   Grade ....   Date ....

School ....   Class Period ....

Pinnie Number	Student Name	Gender	Serve (0-4)	Appropriate Strokes (0-4)	Offensive Tactics (0-4)	Defensive Tactics (0-4)	Total Score (0-16) 12=Competent

8 Floor Hockey

Note: This is a useful assessment. However, because of a small sample size, the ability score for this assessment might not be accurate.

Standard 1:

Demonstrates competency in motor skills and movement patterns needed to perform a variety of physical activities.

Performance Indicator:

Perform the skills and tactics of team sports in a game-like situation.

Assessment Task:

Play a modified game of 3-on-2 floor hockey.

Criteria for Competence (Level 3):

1. Usually uses effective passing, receiving and shooting skills.

2. Player initiating play effectively passes puck and moves to open space to receive a pass 2 times.

3. Usually moves to open space to create a passing lane.

4. Usually moves to intercept puck or make passing difficult for the offensive players.

■ Assessment Rubric:

Level	1. Basic Skills	2. Offensive Skils	3. Movement Wthout the Puck	4. Defensive Skills
4	Consistently uses effective* passing, receiving and shooting skills.	Player initiating play effectively* passes puck and moves to open space to receive a pass 3 times.	Consistently moves to open space with good timing and clear intent to create a passing lane.	Consistently moves to intercept puck or make passing difficult for the offensive players.
3	Usually uses effective passing, receiving and shooting skills.	Player initiating play effectively passes puck and moves to open space to receive a pass 2 times.	Usually moves to open space to create a passing lane.	Usually moves to intercept puck or make passing difficult for the offensive players.
2	Sometimes uses effective passing, receiving and shooting skills.	Player initiating play passes puck and moves to open space to receive a pass 1 time.	Sometimes moves to open space.	Sometimes moves to intercept puck or make passing difficult for the offensive players.
1	Seldom uses effective passing, receiving and shooting skills.	Player initiating play passes puck and never moves to open space to receive a pass.	Seldom moves to open space.	Seldom moves to intercept puck or make passing difficult for the offensive players.
0	Violates safety procedures and/or does not complete the assessment task.			

*Effective is defined as receiving or sending a playable pass, accurate shooting on goal

Scoring: Consistently = 90% or above; Usually = 75% – 89%; Sometimes = 50% –74%; Seldom = below 50%

■ Assessment Protocols:

Directions for Students (Read aloud, verbatim):

- You will play a modified game of 3-on-2 floor hockey, 3 players on offense and 2 players on defense.

- You will be assessed on your ability to:
    a) Use effective passing, receiving and shooting skills.
    b) Move to open space after initiating a pass.
    c) Move to open space to create a pssing lane.
    d) Move to intercept puck or make passing difficult for the offensive players.

- How to start/re-start play: The offensive team will line up behind the center-court line. The center player starts play with a pass to a teammate. The offense will try to move the puck toward the goal and score. Each offensive player will have 3 trials to begin play. Go back to the starting line and begin again if the defense intercepts the puck, you score a goal or the puck goes out of bounds.

Directions for Teachers:

Preparation:

- See the chapter titled Administering & Scoring PE Metrics Assessments for instruction and warm-up.

- Assign students to teams of equally skilled players.

- Teams will play without a goalie.

- Trials will continue until each offensive player has 3 trials to initiate play.

- Each offensive player rotates to the center position on the starting line to initiate 3 plays.

- Make sure that players begin play on or behind center-court line.

Safety:

- Make sure that floor is clean and dry, and that sidelines areas are free from obstacles.

- Enforce safety rules for stick handling.

Equipment/Materials:

- Hockey sticks for each player.

- At least two hockey pucks.

- Goal or 2 cones to mark goal area.

- Numbered pinnies of different colors for offense and defense.

Diagram of Space/Distances:

Use half of a basketball court. Play will begin on or behind center-court line.

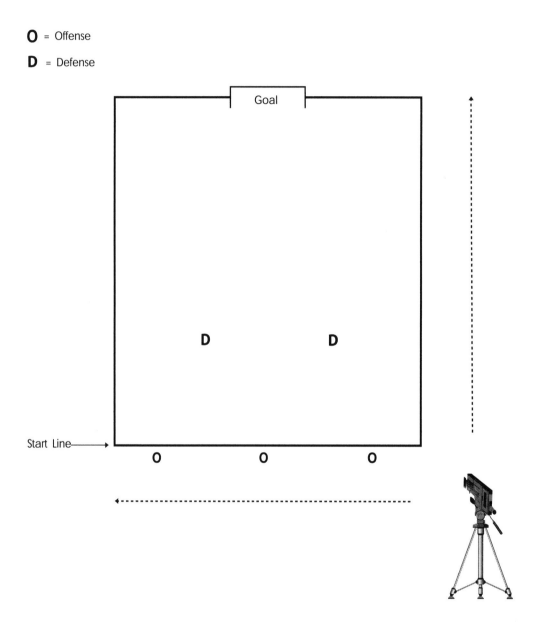

O = Offense

D = Defense

Goal

D   D

Start Line →

O   O   O

Camera Location/Operation:

Place the camera to the side and behind the mid-court line so that the players and the goal can be viewed for the entire distance to be traveled. The beginning line (half-court) should be seen at the left, and the end line should be visible in the viewing screen.

Assessment Score Sheet

PE Teacher _____ Grade _____ Date _____

School _____ Class Period _____

Pinnie Number	Student Name	Gender	Basic Skills (0-4)	Offensive Skills (0-4)	Movement Without the Puck (0-4)	Defensive Skills (0-4) 12=Competent	Total Score (0-16)

8 Grade
Folk Dance

Note: This is a useful assessment. However, because of a small sample size, the ability score for this assessment might not be accurate.

Standard 1:

Demonstrates competency in motor skills and movement patterns needed to perform a variety of physical activities.

Performance Indicator:

Perform specific patterns and sequences in dance and rhythmic activities.

Assessment Task:

Perform a partner or group folk/ethnic/square dance.

Criteria for Competence (Level 3):

1. Consistently performs steps and sequences correctly.
2. Consistently performs to the beat of the music.
3. Consistently synchronizes movements with a partner or group.

■ Assessment Rubric:

Level	1. Steps & Sequences	2. Performs to Beat of the Music	3. Synchronizes Movements With Others
4	Always performs steps and sequences correctly.	Always performs to the beat of the music.	Always synchronizes movements with a partner or group.
3	Consistently performs steps and sequences correctly.	Consistently performs to the beat of the music.	Consistently synchronizes movements with a partner or group.
2	Usually performs steps and sequences correctly.	Usually performs to the beat of the music.	Usually synchronizes movements with a partner or group.
1	Sometimes or seldom performs steps and sequences correctly.	Sometimes or seldom performs to the beat of the music.	Sometimes or seldom synchronizes movements with a partner or group.
0	Violates safety procedures and/or does not complete the assessment task.		

Scoring: Always = 100%; Consistently = 90% – 99%; Usually = 75% – 89%; Sometimes or Seldom = below 75%

■ Assessment Protocols:

Directions for Students (Read aloud, verbatim):

- You will be asked to perform a folk/ethnic/square dance.

- You will be assessed on your ability to:
    a) Perform the steps and sequences of the dance correctly.
    b) Move to the beat of the music.
    c) Synchronize movements with a partner or group.

- You will perform in groups, using the formation required for the dance.

Directions for Teachers:

Preparation:

- See the chapter titled Administering & Scoring PE Metrics Assessments for instruction and warm-up.

- Select an age-appropriate dance from those that students have been taught and have practiced. The dance selected should include at least 3 different steps.

- Do not coach or call the steps during the assessment.

- Camera placement might vary, depending on the dance. Place the camera in a position where you can see students' numbers and the entire dance sequence clearly. The camera on the diagram is positioned for a square dance.

- Students in groups of no more than 8 should be spaced so that each can be seen clearly.

- Attach the written directions to the dance to the scoring sheet.

Safety:

- Dance area is clean and dry, free from obstruction(s), with clear perimeter to the dance area.

Equipment/Materials:

- CD/tape player and CD/tape for the dance.

- Numbered pinnies.

Diagram of Space/Distances:

△ = Cone

D = Dancer

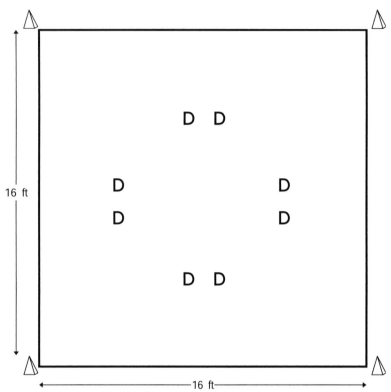

16 ft

16 ft

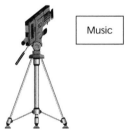

Music

Camera Location/Operation:
The camera should be located at the corner of the dance area and elevated so that all dancers can be viewed (may vary depending on dance). The cones marking the dance area must be visible on the viewing screen. Music source should be placed close enough to the camera to be recorded.

Assessment Score Sheet

PE Teacher _____   Grade _____   Date _____

School _____   Class Period _____

Pinnie Number	Student Name	Gender	Steps & Sequences (0-4)	Performs to Beat of the Music (0-4)	Synchronizes Movements With Others (0-4)	Total Score (0-12) 9=Competent

8 Line Dance

Grade

Standard 1:

Demonstrates competency in motor skills and movement patterns needed to perform a variety of physical activities.

Performance Indicator:

Perform specific patterns and sequences in dance and rhythmic activities.

Assessment Task:

Perform a line dance.

Criteria for Competence (Level 3):

1. Consistently performs steps and sequences correctly.
2. Consistently performs to the beat of the music.

■ Assessment Rubric:

Level	1. Steps & Sequences	2. Moves to the Beat of the Music
4	Always performs steps and sequences correctly.	Always performs to the beat of the music.
3	Consistently performs steps and sequences correctly.	Consistently performs to the beat of the music.
2	Usually performs steps and sequences correctly.	Usually performs to the beat of the music.
1	Sometimes or seldom performs steps and sequences correctly.	Sometimes or seldom performs to the beat of the music.
0	Violates safety procedures and/or does not complete the assessment task.	

Scoring: Always = 100%; Consistently = 90% – 99% ; Usually = 75% – 89%; Sometimes or Seldom = below 75%

■ Assessment Protocols:

Directions for Students (Read aloud, verbatim):

- You will be asked to perform a line dance.

- You will be assessed on your ability to:
    a) Perform the steps and sequences of the dance correctly.
    b) Move to the beat of the music.

Directions for Teachers:

Preparation:

- See the chapter titled Administering & Scoring PE Metrics Assessments for instruction and warm-up.

- Select an age-appropriate dance from those that students have been taught and have practiced.

- The dance should include at least 4 different steps (e.g., kick ball change, grapevine and touch, shuffle).

- Attach written directions for the dance to the scoring sheet.

Safety:

- Dance area is clean and dry, free from obstruction(s), with clear perimeter around the dance area.

Equipment/Materials:

- CD/tape player.

- CD or tape for the dance.

- Numbered pinnies.

Diagram of Space/Distances:

One line of four students can dance at one time. Place camera so that you can see all of the dancers throughout the entire dance.

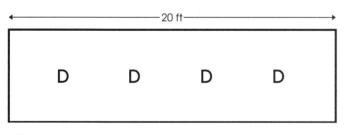

D = Dancer

Camera Location/Operation:

The camera can be placed in front of the dancers so that all 4 can be seen in the viewing screen. Be sure you can see the dancers' entire body, including the feet. Be sure dancers stay in camera view when making sideways movements. The music source must be close enough to the camera so that the music can also be recorded.

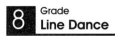 Grade
Line Dance

Assessment Score Sheet

PE Teacher _____ Grade _____ Date _____

School _____ Class Period _____

Pinnie Number	Student Name	Gender	Steps & Sequences (0-4)	Beat of the Music (0-4)	Total Score (0-8) 6=Competent

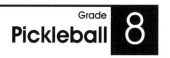

Note: This is a useful assessment. However, because of a small sample size, the ability score for this assessment might not be accurate.

Standard 1:

Demonstrates competency in motor skills and movement patterns needed to perform a variety of physical activities.

Performance Indicator:

Perform the skills and tactics of dual competitive sports in a game-like situation.

Assessment Task:

Play a competitive game of singles pickleball.

Criteria for Competence (Level 3):

1. Uses a legal serve to place the ball into opponent's service area for at least 8 out of 10 serves.

2. Usually chooses appropriate stroke (e.g., forehand, backhand, volley).

3. Usually uses an offensive shot to hit the ball away from opponent to open space.

4. Usually moves to home base and ready position following strokes.

■ Assessment Rubric:

Level	1. Serve	2. Appropriate Strokes	3. Offensive Tactics	4. Defensive Tactics
4	Uses a legal serve to place the ball into opponent's service area for 10 out of 10 serves.	Consistently chooses appropriate stroke.	Consistently uses an offensive shot to hit the ball away from opponent to open space.	Consistently moves to home base and ready position following strokes.
3	Uses a legal serve to place the ball into opponent's service area for at least 8 out of 10 serves.	Usually chooses appropriate stroke.	Usually uses an offensive shot to hit the ball away from opponent to open space.	Usually moves to home base and ready position following strokes.
2	Uses a legal serve to place the ball into opponent's service area for at least 6 out of 10 serves.	Sometimes chooses appropriate stroke.	Sometimes uses an offensive shot to hit the ball away from opponent to open space.	Sometimes moves to home base and ready position following strokes.
1	Uses a legal serve to place the ball into opponent's service area for 5 or fewer out of 10 serves.	Seldom chooses appropriate stroke.	Seldom uses an offensive shot to hit the ball away from opponent to open space.	Seldom moves to home base and ready position following strokes.
0	Violates safety procedures and/or does not complete the assessment task.			

Scoring: Consistently = 90% or above; Usually = 75% – 89%; Sometimes = 50% –74%; Seldom = below 50%

■ **Assessment Protocols:**

Directions for Students (Read aloud, verbatim):

- You will play a competitive singles game of pickleball.

- You will be assessed on your ability to:
    a) Use a legal serve to place the ball into opponent's service area.
    b) Select a forehand, backhand and volley appropriately.
    c) Use an offensive shot to hit the ball away from opponent to open space.
    d) Move to home base and ready position following all strokes.

- Start play: Play will begin with service by the player on the side opposite the camera, who will serve 10 times.

- Alternate right and left service area on each serve. Call line violations on your side of the court.

- Play on each serve will continue until the point is won/lost. No score is to be recorded.

- Change sides and server at the completion of 10 serves.

Directions for Teachers:

- See the chapter titled Administering & Scoring PE Metrics Assessments for instruction and warm-up.

- Select players of similar ability as opponents.

- No score is to be kept.

- So that skills can be viewed from the same angle for both players, play should continue until one player completes 10 serves (with play after each serve continuing until the point is ended).

- Change sides and server at the completion of 10 serves.

- All rules (with the exception of scoring) should apply. Players will call line violations on their respective sides of the court.

Safety:

- Courts are to be dry and free of obstruction, with adequate out-of-bounds space surrounding all sides.

Equipment/Materials:

- Nets, standards and floor markings for each court. Usually, a badminton court is appropriate for pickleball.

- Pickleball paddles and at least 2 balls for each court.

- Numbered pinnies.

Diagram of Space/Distances:

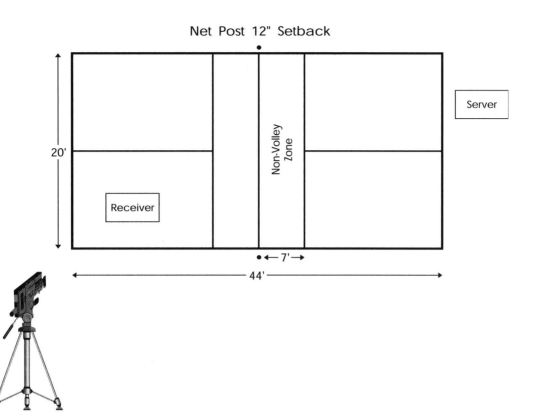

Net Post 12" Setback

Server

Non-Volley Zone

Receiver

20'

● ← 7' →

44'

Camera Location/Operation:

The camera should be placed at the corner of the court so that both end lines and sidelines can be seen at the edge of the viewing screen. Camera should be placed so that all play of both players can be viewed without moving/panning during play or interfering with the movement of the receiver.

Assessment Score Sheet

PE Teacher _____ Grade _____ Date _____

School _____ Class Period _____

Pinnie Number	Student Name	Gender	Serve (0-4)	Appropriate Strokes (0-4)	Offensive Tactics (0-4)	Defensive Tactics (0-4)	Total Score (0-16) 12=Competent

Standard 1:

Demonstrates competency in motor skills and movement patterns needed to perform a variety of physical activities.

Performance Indicator:

Perform the skills and tactics of team sports in a game-like situation.

Assessment Task:

Play a modified game of 3-on-2 soccer.

Criteria for Competence (Level 3):

1. Usually uses effective passing, receiving and shooting skills.
2. Player initiating play effectively passes ball and moves to appropriate space to receive a pass 2 times.
3. Usually moves to open space to create a passing lane.
4. Usually moves to intercept ball or make passing difficult for the offensive players.

■ Assessment Rubric:

Level	1. Basic Skills	2. Offensive Skills	3. Movement Without the Ball	4. Defensive Skills
4	Consistently uses effective* passing, receiving and shooting skills.	Player initiating play effectively* passes ball and moves to open space to receive a pass 3 times.	Consistently moves to open space, with good timing and clear intent to create a passing lane.	Consistently moves to intercept ball or make passing difficult for the offensive players.
3	Usually uses effective passing, receiving and shooting skills.	Player initiating play effectively* passes ball and moves to open space to receive a pass 2 times.	Usually moves to open space to create a passing lane.	Usually moves to intercept ball or make passing difficult for the offensive players.
2	Sometimes uses effective passing, receiving and shooting skills.	Player initiating play passes ball and moves to open space to receive a pass 1 time.	Sometimes moves to open space.	Sometimes moves to intercept ball or make passing difficult for the offensive players.
1	Seldom uses effective passing, receiving and shooting skills.	Player initiating play passes ball and never moves to open space to receive a pass.	Seldom moves to open space.	Seldom moves to intercept ball or make passing difficult for the offensive players.
0	Violates safety procedures and/or does not complete the assessment task.			

*Effective is defined as receiving or sending a playable pass, accurate shooting on goal.

Scoring: Scoring: Consistently = 90% or above; Usually = 75% – 89%; Sometimes = 50% – 74%; Seldom = below 50%

■ Assessment Protocols:

Directions for Students (Read aloud, verbatim):

- You will play a modified 3-on-2 game of soccer; 3 players on offense and 2 players on defense.

- You will be assessed on your ability to:

    a) Use appropriate passing, receiving and shooting skills.

    b) Move to open space after initiating a pass.

    c) Move to open space to create a passing lane.

    d) Move to intercept ball or make passing difficult for the offensive players.

- How to start/restart play: The offensive team will line up behind the center line of the field. The center player starts play with a pass to a teammate. The ofense will try to move the ball toward the goal and score. Each offensive player will have 3 trials to begin play. Go back to the starting line and begin again if the defense intercepts the ball, you score a goal or the ball goes out of bounds.

- Defensive players start at midfield.

Directions for Teachers:

- See the chapter titled Administering & Scoring PE Metrics Assessments for instruction and warm-up.

- Assign students to teams of equally skilled players.

- Teams will play without a goalie.

- Trials will continue until an offensive player has 3 trials to initiate play.

- Each offensive player rotates to the center position on the starting line to initiate 3 plays.

- Make sure that players begin play on or behind center field line.

Safety:

- Make sure that fields and sideline areas are free from obstruction and hazardous objects, are level (without holes) and are mowed.

Equipment/Materials:

- Lined outdoor field (use a proportionally modified half soccer field).

- At least three regulation soccer balls to keep the game going.

- Goal or 2 cones to mark goal area.

- 4 cones to mark corners of playing area.

- Personal safety equipment: shin guards.

- Numbered pinnies of different colors for offense and defense.

Diagram of Space/Distances:

Use one half of a regulation soccer field. Use a regulation-size goal.

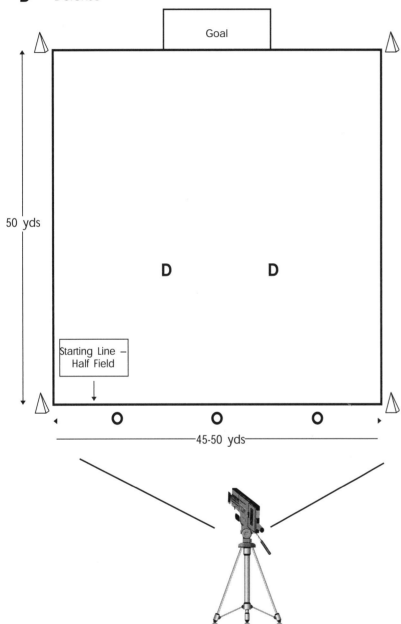

△ = Cone

O = Offense

D = Defense

Camera Location/Operation:

The camera should be behind the starting line so that both sides of the field and the goal can be seen at the top and bottom of the viewing screen; the sides of the field can be seen at the side of the viewing screen.

Assessment Score Sheet

PE Teacher _____ Grade _____ Date _____

School _____ Class Period _____

Pinnie Number	Student Name	Gender	Basic Skills (0-4)	Offensive Skills (0-4)	Movement Without Ball (0-4)	Defensive Skills (0-4)	Total Score (0-16) 12=Competent

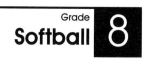
Note: This is a useful assessment. However, because of a small sample size, the ability score for this assessment might not be accurate.

Standard 1:

Demonstrates competency in motor skills and movement patterns needed to perform a variety of physical activities.

Performance Indicator:

Perform the skills and tactics of team sports in a game-like situation.

Assessment Task:

Field a ground ball, throw a catchable ball and catch a catchable ball.

Criteria for Competence (Level 3):

1. Cleanly fields a catchable* ground ball.
2. Transitions from fielding to throwing using a smooth, continuous motion on 2 trials.
3. Throws a catchable ball to first base ahead of runner on 2 of 3 trials.
4. Catches a catchable* ball thrown from 2nd-base player.

■ Assessment Rubric:

Level	1. Fields Ground Ball	2. Transitions to Throw	3. Throws to 1st Base	4. Catches a Catchable* Ball at 1st Base Thrown From 2nd Base
4	Charges forward to cleanly field a playable ground ball.	Transitions from fielding to throwing using a smooth and continuous motion on all 3 trials.	Throws a catchable ball to 1st base ahead of runner.	Catches, with glove extended toward ball, a catchable ball thrown from 2nd-base player.
3	Cleanly fields a playable ground ball.	Transitions from fielding to throwing using a smooth and continuous motion on 2 trials.	Throws a catchable ball to 1st base ahead of runner on 2 of 3 trials.	Catches a chatchable* ball thrown from 2nd- base player.
2	Fields a playable ground ball with bobble before control.	Transitions from fielding to throwing using a smooth and continuous motion on 1 trial.	Throws a catchable ball to 1st base ahead of runner on 1 of 3 trials.	Bobbles but catches a catchable ball thrown from 2nd-base player.
1	Drops or misses a playable ground ball.	Does not transition from fielding to throwing using a smooth and continuous motion on any trial.	Does not throw a catchable ball to 1st base ahead of runner on any trial.	Drops a catchable ball from 2nd-base player.
0	Violates safety procedures and/or does not complete the assessment task.			

*Give additional trial if the throw from 2nd to 1st base is uncatchable, as determined by the teacher.

■ **Assessment Protocols:**

Directions for Students (Read aloud, verbatim):

- You will be fielding a ground ball at 2nd base, throwing to 1st base and catching at 1st base.

- You will be working in groups of 3 to complete the drill.

- You will be assessed on your ability to:
    a) Field a catchable ground ball thrown from home plate to near 2nd-base.
    b) Throw a catchable ball to 1st base.
    c) Catch at 1st base a catchable ball thrown from 2nd-base player.

- The teacher or a designated thrower (trained to throw a ground ball from home plate to near 2nd base consistently) will throw a ground ball from home plate toward the fielder (#2).

- On my command, the runner (#1) will run from home plate to tag 1st base.

- The fielder will field the ball and throw to the 1st base player (#3).

- You will rotate counterclockwise after 3 trials are completed. The runner becomes the 1st base player, the 1st base player becomes the fielder, the fielder goes to home plate and becomes the runner.

- Repeat the drill until all players have completed 3 trials in each position.

Directions for Teachers:
Preparation:

- See the chapter titled Administering & Scoring PE Metrics Assessments for instruction and warm-up.

- Assign students to groups of equal skills.

- Serve as "thrower" or train a student thrower who can consistently throw a ground ball to near 2nd base. The ball should be a rolling ball rather than a bouncing ball.

- Place the fielder in 2nd-base position, and another player at 1st base.

- Give signal to runner as ground ball is thrown.

- If a student does not have the opportunity to receive at least 3 catchable balls in each position, give him/her another opportunity.

- After players complete the assessment, rotate them to help retrieve passed balls (2 behind the fielder, 1 behind 1st base).

Safety:

- Make sure that fields are free from obstruction, and are level (without holes) and mowed.

Equipment/Materials:

- One-half of a softball diamond.

- Home plate and 2 bases.

- Gloves for all players.

- Regulation-size softballs.

Diagram of Space/Distances:

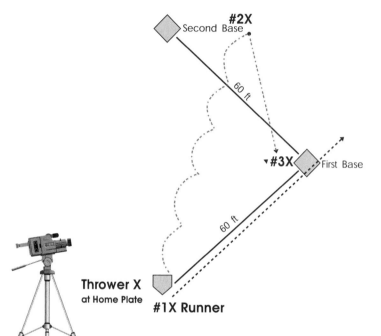

----------- = Ball Path

----------- = Path of Runner

_____ = Baseline

#2X and **#3X** = Players on Field

#1X = Runner

#2X
Second Base

60 ft

#3X First Base

60 ft

Thrower X
at Home Plate
#1X Runner

Camera Location/Operation:

The camera can be placed to the left of home plate so that 1st base and 2nd base can be seen fully on the viewing screen.

Assessment Score Sheet

PE Teacher _____   Grade _____   Date _____

School _____   Class Period _____

Pinnie Number	Student Name	Gender	Field (0-12)			Transition (0-12)			Throw (0-12)			Catch (0-12)			Total Score (0-48) 36=Competent
			1	2	3	1	2	3	1	2	3	1	2	3	

Standard 1:

Demonstrates competency in motor skills and movement patterns needed to perform a variety of physical activities.

Performance Indicator:

Perform the skills and tactics of team sports in a game-like situation.

Assessment Task:

Play a modified game of 3-on-2 team handball.

Criteria for Competence (Level 3):

1. Usually uses effective passing, receiving and shooting skills.

2. Player initiating play effectively passes ball and moves to open space to receive a pass 2 times.

3. Usually moves to open space to create a passing lane.

4. Usually moves to intercept ball or make passing difficult for the offensive players.

■ Assessment Rubric:

Level	1. Basic Skills	2. Offensive Skills	3. Movement Without the Ball	4. Defensive Tactics
4	Consistently uses effective* passing, receiving and shooting skills.	Player initiating play effectively* passes ball and moves to open space to receive a pass 3 times.	Consistently moves to open space with good timing and clear intent to create a passing lane.	Consistently moves to intercept ball or make passing difficult for the offensive players.
3	Usually uses effective passing, receiving and shooting skills.	Player initiating play effectively passes ball and moves to open space to receive a pass 2 times.	Ususally moves to open space to create a passing lane.	Usually moves to intercept ball or make passing difficult for the offensive players.
2	Sometimes uses effective passing, receiving and shooting skills.	Player initiating play passes ball and moves to open space to receive a pass 1 time.	Sometimes moves to open space.	Sometimes moves to intercept ball or make passing difficult for the offensive players.
1	Seldom uses effective passing, receiving and shooting skills.	Player initiating play passes ball and never moves to open space to receive a pass.	Seldom moves to open space.	Seldom moves to intercept ball or make passing difficult for the offensive players.
0	Violates safety procedures and/or does not complete the assessment task.			

*Effective is defined as catching or sending a receivable pass, accurate shooting on goal

Scoring: Consistently = 90% or above; Usually = 75% – 89%; Sometimes = 50% – 74%; Seldom = below 50%

■ **Assessment Protocols:**

Directions for Students (Read aloud, verbatim):

- You will play a modified 3-on-2 game of team handball, 3 players on offense and 2 players on defense.

- You will be assessed on your ability to:
    a) Use effective passing, receiving and shooting skills.
    b) Move to open space after initiating a pass.
    c) Move to open space to create a passing lane.
    d) Move to intercept ball or make passing difficult for the offensive players.

- How to start/restart play: The offensive team will line up behind the center-court line. The center player starts play with a pass to a teammate. The offense will try to move the ball toward the goal and score. Each offensive player will have 3 trials to begin play. Go back to the starting line and begin again if the defense intercepts the ball, you score a goal or the ball goes out of bounds.

Directions for Teachers:

- See the chapter titled Administering & Scoring PE Metrics Assessments for instruction and warm-up.

- Assign students to teams of equally skilled players.

- Teams will play without a goalie.

- Trials will continue until each offensive player has 3 trials to initiate play.

- Each offensive player rotates to the center position on the starting line to initiate 3 plays.

- Make sure that players begin play on or behind center-court line.

Safety:

- Courts are to be dry and free of obstruction, with adequate out-of-bounds space surrounding all sides.

Equipment/Materials:

- One-half of a gymnasium.

- Team handball.

- Goal or 2 cones to mark goal area.

- Numbered pinnies of different colors for offense and defense.

Diagram of Space/Distances:

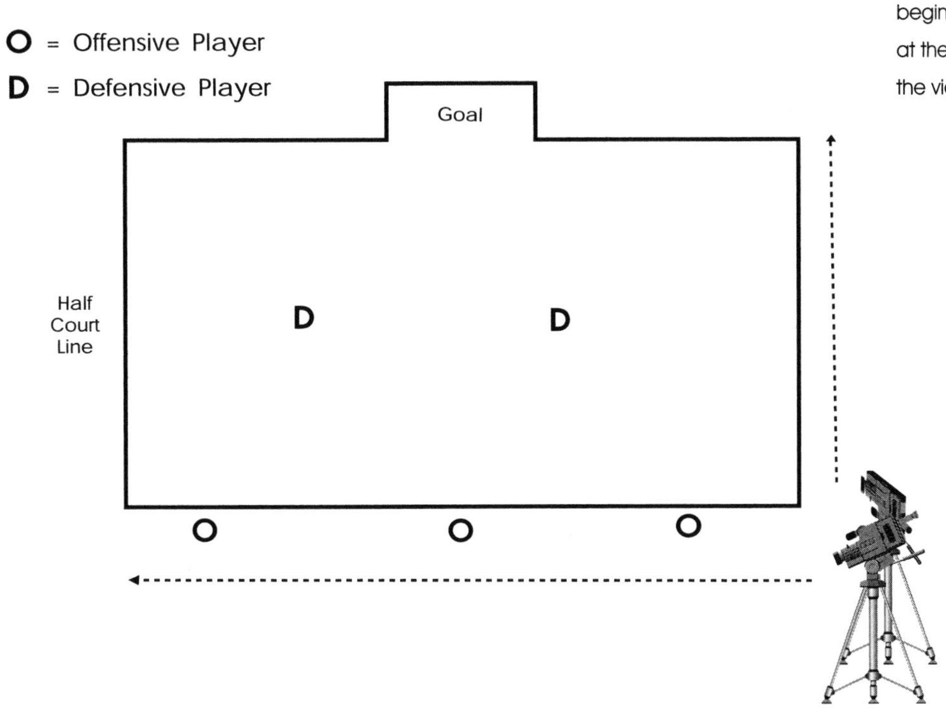

Camera Location/Operation:

The camera should be placed to the side and behind the midcourt line so that the players and the goal can be viewed for the entire distance to be traveled. The beginning line (half court) should be seen at the left and the end line at the right of the viewing screen.

O = Offensive Player

D = Defensive Player

Goal

Half
Court
Line

D   D

O   O   O

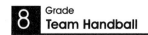

Assessment Score Sheet

PE Teacher _____   Grade _____   Date _____

School _____   Class Period _____

Pinnie Number	Student Name	Gender	Basic Skills (0-4)	Offensive Skills (0-4)	Movement Without the Ball (0-4)	Defensive Skills (0-4)	Total Score (0-16) 12=Competent

Traverse Climbing

Standard 1:

Demonstrates competency in motor skills and movement patterns needed to perform a variety of physical activities.

Performance Indicator:

Perform basic skills in adventure/outdoor activities.

Assessment Task:

Traverse a horizontal climbing wall.

Criteria for Competence (Level 3):

1. Uusually meets criteria for proper technique:
   a) Faces wall.
   b) Maintains 3 points of contact.
   c) Keeps hips close to wall.
2. Usually uses legs to support weight and uses handholds for balance.
3. Executes well-planned movements, with 1 crossover.
4. Completes 20-foot traverse, with no more than 1 fall.

■ Assessment Rubric:

Level	1. Proper Technique	2. Legs for Support & Hands for Balance	3. Crossover	4. Completes 20-foot Traverse
4	Consistently meets criteria for proper technique.	Consistently uses legs for support and handholds for balance.	Executes well-planned movements, with no cross-over.	Completes 20-foot traverse without falling.
3	Usually meets criteria for proper technique.	Usually uses legs for support and handholds for balance.	Executes well-planned movements, with one crossover.	Completes 20-foot traverse with no more than 1 fall.
2	Sometimes meets criteria for proper technique.	Sometimes uses legs for support and handholds for balance.	Executes 2 crossovers.	Completes 20-foot traverse with no more than 2 falls.
1	Seldom meets criteria for proper technique.	Seldom uses legs for support and handholds for balance.	Executes more than 2 crossovers.	Completes 20-foot traverse with 3 or more falls.
0	Violates safety procedures and/or does not complete the assessment task.			

Scoring: Consistently = 90% or above; Usually = 75% – 89%; Sometimes = 50% –74%; Seldom = below 50%

■ Assessment Protocols:

Directions for Students (Read aloud, verbatim):

- You will be asked to traverse a climbing wall for a distance of 20 feet in your preferred direction. Your partner will be the spotter and will follow closely, with hands up and knees bent, ready to break your fall, if necessary.

- You will be assessed on your ability to:
    a) Maintain 3 points of contact, face wall, keep hips close to the wall.
    b) Use your legs to support your weight and use your hands for balance.
    c) Execute well planned movements without crossovers.
    d) Complete the 20 foot traverse without falling.

- Follow all safety rules.

Directions for Teachers:
Preparation:

- See the chapter titled Administering & Scoring PE Metrics Assessments for instruction and warm-up.

- Assign partners of equal size, weight and ability.

- Film one student at a time completing the traverse climb. Film all students traveling in one preferred direction (e.g., left to right), then move camera to other side for students who prefer to travel in the other direction (e.g., right to left).

- Students should not be coached or given any instruction or encouragement while they are climbing.

- If a student falls during the traverse, he/she should resume the traverse climb at that spot.

Safety:

- Student spotter should be close to partner, with hands up and knees bent, ready to break the fall.

- The teacher should check the wall's safety.

- All students should remove objects from clothing, neck and fingers.

- Secure eyeglasses.

- Instructions about objectives, safety procedures and hazards must be clearly understood.

- Place protective mats on the floor along the climbing wall, extending at least 5 feet from the wall.

Equipment/Materials:

- 20' X 8' horizontal climbing wall.

- Mats along wall and extending at least 5 feet from the wall.

Diagram of Space/Distances:

C = Climber starting position

S = Spotter starting position

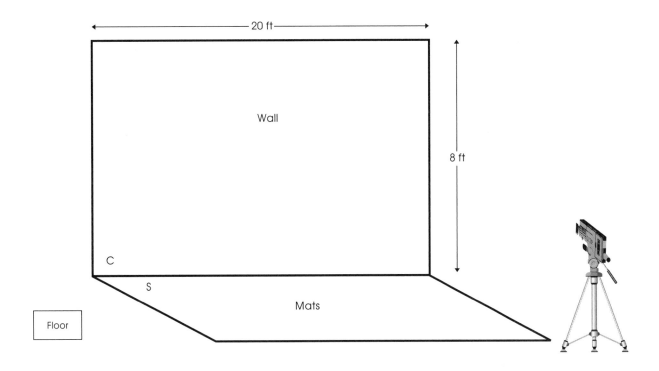

Camera Location/Operation:

Place the camera at an angle to the wall near the end toward which the climber is traversing so that moves can be clearly seen and communication between climber and spotter can be heard.

Assessment Score Sheet

PE Teacher _____ Grade _____ Date _____

School _____ Class Period _____

Pinnie Number	Student Name	Gender	Points of Contact (0-4)	Leg Support/ Hand Balance (0-4)	Crossover (0-4)	Complete 20-ft. Traverse 1 Direction (0-4)	Total Score (0-16) 12=Competent

Standard 1:

Demonstrates competency in motor skills and movement patterns needed to perform a variety of physical activities.

Performance Indicator:

Perform the skills and tactics of team sports in a game-like situation.

Assessment Task:

Play 3-on-3 modified game of Ultimate Frisbee®.

Criteria for Competence (Level 3):

1. Usually uses effective passing and receiving skills.
2. Usually in a position to support a teammate on offense by moving to an open space.
3. Usually marks an opponent defensively by moving with and staying between the same opponent and the goal.

■ Assessment Rubric:

Level	1. Basic Skills	2. Offense	3. Defense
4	Consistently uses effective* passing and receiving skills.	Consistently in a position to support a teammate on offense by moving to open space.	Consistently marks an opponent defensively by moving with and staying between the same opponent and the goal.
3	Usually uses effective passing and receiving skills.	Usually in a position to support a teammate on offense by moving to open space.	Usually marks an opponent defensively by moving with and staying between the same opponent and the goal.
2	Sometimes uses effective passing and receiving skills.	Sometimes in a position to support a teammate on offense by moving to open space.	Sometimes marks an opponent defensively by moving with and staying between the same opponent and the goal.
1	Seldom uses effective passing and receiving skills.	Seldom in a position to support a teammate on offense by moving to open space.	Seldom marks an opponent defensively by moving with and staying between the same opponent and the goal.
0	Violates safety procedures and/or does not complete the assessment task.		

*Effective is defined as sending or receiving a playable pass.

Scoring: Consistently = 90% or above; Usually = 75% – 89%; Sometimes = 50% –74%; Seldom = below 50%

■ Assessment Protocols:

Directions for Students (Read aloud, verbatim):

- You will be asked to play a 3-on-3 modified game of Ultimate Frisbee®.

- You will be assessed on your ability to:

    a) Pass and receive effectively.

    b) Position yourself to support a teammate on offense by moving to open space.

    c) Mark an opponent defensively by moving with and staying between the same opponent and the goal.

Game Rules

- Start/re-start play: At the beginning of play and after each goal, each team lines up on its respective goal line and one team throws the disk to the other team. When play stops (e.g., when disk hits the ground, 10-second count, thrower catches own throw or hands disk to teammates), restart play by touching the disk to the ground and announcing "In play."

- You will play two 5-minute periods, alternating possessions.

Directions for Teachers:

- See the chapter titled Administering & Scoring PE Metrics Assessments for instruction and warm-up.

- Assign students to teams of equally skilled players.

Safety:

- Make sure that fields are free from obstruction and hazardous objects, and are level (without holes) and mowed.

- Use a standard-weight disk in good condition (no rough edges or cracks).

Equipment/Materials:

- 50' x 50' outdoor playing field.

- 2 Frisbees®.

- Numbered pinnies of different colors for offense and defense.

Diagram of Space/Distances:

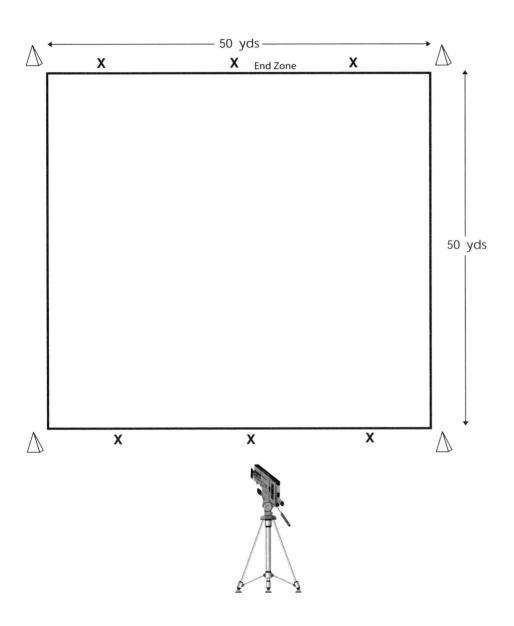

= Cone

X = Players

50 yds

End Zone

50 yds

Camera Location/Operation:

The camera so that you can see the entire playing field. For most cameras that means behind, and somewhat in back of, one of the end zones in the corner, with an open wide angle.

Assessment Score Sheet

PE Teacher _____   Grade _____   Date _____

School _____   Class Period _____

Pinnie Number	Student Name	Gender	Basic Skills (0-4)	Offense (0-4)	Defense (0-4)	Total Score (0-12) 8=Competent

Standard 1:

Demonstrates competency in motor skills and movement patterns needed to perform a variety of physical activities.

Performance Indicator:

Perform the skills and tactics of team sports in a game-like situation.

Assessment Task:

Overhead and forearm-pass a tossed ball to a target player.

Criteria for Competence (Level 3):

1. Executes a forearm pass from a playable tossed ball on at least 4 of 5 trials, meeting the following criteria:

   a) Legal forearm pass.

   b) 10-15 feet in height (3-5 feet higher than net) on same side of court.

2. Target player catches a pass that meets both criteria in #1 within 7-foot square 3 out of 5 trials.

3. Executes an overhead pass from a playable tossed ball on at least 4 of 5 trials, meeting the following criteria:

   a) Legal overhead pass.

   b) 10-15 feet in height (3-5 feet higher than net) on same side of court.

4. Target player catches a pass that meets both criteria in #3 within 7-foot square 3 out of 5 trials.

- ■ **Assessment Rubric:**

Level	1. Forearm Pass Criteria	2. Forearm Pass Accuracy	3. Overhead Pass Criteria	4. Overhead Pass Accuracy
4	Meets both criteria on all 5 trials.	Target player catches pass that meets criteria within 7-foot square 4 out of 5 trials.	Meets both criteria on all 5 trials.	Target player catches ball that meets criteria within 7-foot square 4 out of 5 trials.
3	Executes overhead pass on 4 out of 5 trials, meeting the criteria: a. Legal pass. b. 10-15 feet in height.	Target player catches pass that meets criteria within 7-foot square 3 out of 5 trials.	Executes overhead pass on 4 out of 5 trials, meeting the criteria: c. Legal pass. d. 10-15 feet in height.	Target player catches pass that meets criteria within 7-foot square 3 out of 5 trials.
2	Meets both criteria on 3 out of 5 trials.	Target player catches pass that meets criteria within 7-foot square 2 out of 5 trials.	Meets both criteria on 3 out of 5 trials.	Target player catches pass that meets criteria within 7-foot square 2 out of 5 trials.
1	Meets both criteria on 2 or fewer out of 5 trials.	Target player catches pass that meets criteria within 7-foot square 1 or fewer times out of 5 trials.	Meets both criteria on 2 or fewer out of 5 trials.	Target player catches pass that meets criteria within 7-foot square 1 or fewer out of 5 trials.
0	Violates safety procedures and/or does not complete the assessment task.			

■ Assessment Protocols:

Directions for Students (Read aloud, verbatim):

- You will be assessed on your ability execute a forearm pass and overhead pass at least 3 to 5 feet higher than the net so that the target player doesn't have to go out of the square to catch the ball. You will have 5 opportunities for each type of pass.

- Forearm pass: The tosser will toss you an overhand rainbow toss across the net. You will use a forearm pass to send the ball to a target player at the net. The pass must go at least 3 to 5 feet higher than the net and must be catchable by the receiver standing within the square.

- Overhead pass: You will receive an underhand-tossed ball from the back of your side of the court. You will stand in a center position at the net and use an overhead pass to send the ball to the target player on the same side of the net. The pass must go at least 3 to 5 feet higher than the net and must be catchable by the receiver standing in the square.

Directions for Teachers:

- See the chapter titled Administering & Scoring PE Metrics Assessments for instruction and warm-up.

- Passer is located in the center back for the forearm pass and in the center front for the overhead pass.

- Location of "tosser" for the forearm pass is behind the spiking line on opposite side of net from passer. The person tossing the ball from across the net should try to emulate a rainbow serve and put the ball as close as possible to the player being assessed.

- Location of "tosser" for the overhead pass is from the center back position. The toss should be underhand and simulate a high forearm pass.

- The toss is crucial in this assessment. A skilled tosser is essential.

- If a toss is not close to the player (passer), the tosser should re-toss the ball.

- Repeat the directions if necessary before beginning the second part of the assessment for the overhead pass.

Safety:

- Floor is to be dry, clean and clear of obstacles at least beyond the boundary of the court.

Equipment/Materials:

- Volleyball court.

- Regulation leather volleyballs.

- Numbered pinnies.

- Use tape or chalk to mark 7-foot squares in the center and left front line position of one side of the court. The edge of the square should touch the center line.

Diagram of Space/Distances:

Forearm Pass

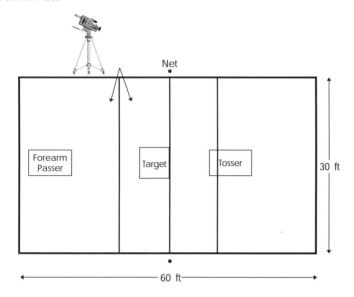

Camera Location/Operation:

The camera should be placed so that the entire playing area on the receiving side of the net can be seen on the viewing screen. Both passer and target receiver must be seen without moving the camera.

Overhead Pass

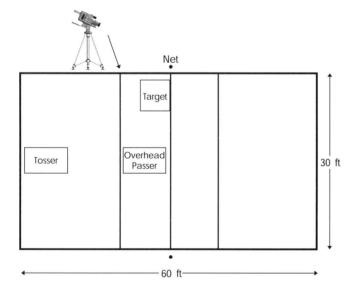

Camera Location/Operation:

The camera must be placed so the tosser, passer and the target receiver can be seen without moving the camera.

Assessment Score Sheet

PE Teacher _____   Grade _____   Date _____

School _____   Class Period _____

Pinnie Number	Student Name	Gender	Forearm Pass Criteria (0-4)	Forearm Pass Accuracy (0-4)	Overhead Pass Criteria (0-4)	Overhead Pass Accuracy (0-4)	Total Score (0-16) 12=Competent

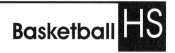

Standard 1:

Demonstrates competency in motor skills and movement patterns needed to perform a variety of physical activities.

Performance Indicator:

Demonstrate competence in team court sports.

Assessment Task:

Play a 3-on-3 half-court basketball game.

Criteria for Competence (Level 3):

1. Usually uses effective ball skills (dribbling, passing, catching, shooting) with good technique and control.

2. Usually moves to get open to an appropriate space to receive/send a pass.

3. Usually in a position to use individual defensive skills (guarding and blocking).

4. Usually moves easily into a team defensive position (player-to-player, zone).

■ Assessment Rubric:

Level	1. Ball Skills	2. Offensive Play	3. Individual Defensive Play	4. Team Defense
4	Consistently uses effective ball skills with good technique and control.	Consistently moves to get open to an appropriate space to receive/send a pass.	Consistently in a position to use individual defensive skills (guarding and blocking).	Consistently moves easily into a team defensive position (player-to-player, zone).
3	Usually uses effective ball skills with good technique and control (dribbling, passing, catching, shooting).	Usually moves to get open to an appropriate space to receive/send a pass.	Usually in a position to use individual defensive skills (guarding players and blocking shots).	Usually moves easily into a team defensive position (player-to-player, zone).
2	Sometimes uses effective ball skills with good technique and control.	Sometimes moves to get open to an appropriate space to receive/send a pass.	Sometimes in a position to use individual defensive skills (guarding and blocking).	Sometimes moves easily into a team defensive position (player-to-player, zone).
1	Seldom uses effective ball skills with good technique and control.	Seldom moves to get open to an appropriate space to receive/send a pass.	Seldom in position to use individual defensive skills (guarding and blocking).	Seldom moves easily into a team defensive position (player-to- player, zone).
0	Violates safety procedures and/or does not complete the assessment task.			

Scoring: Consistently = 90% or above; Usually = 75% – 89%; Sometimes = 50% –74%; Seldom = below 50%

■ Assessment Protocols:

Directions for Students (Read aloud, verbatim):

- You will be asked to play a modified game of basketball with three people on a side using a half court for 8 minutes.

- Modified rules of half-court basketball will be used.

- The game will start at half-court and resume after each score by the non-scoring team putting the ball in play at half court (no make, take it). You will be asked to call your own out-of-bounds and rules violations, and keep score.

- You will be assessed on your ability to:
    a)   Use effective ball skills with good technique and control (dribbling, passing, catching, shooting).
    b)   Move to get open to an appropriate space to receive/send a pass.
    c)   Move to a position to use individual defensive skills (guarding and blocking).
    d)   Move easily into a team defensive position (player-to-player, zone).

Directions for Teachers:
Preparation:

- See the chapter titled Administering & Scoring PE Metrics Assessments for instruction and warm-up.

- Assign students to be tested to a team of three students. Try to assign students of *relatively* equal ability to a team, and have students play a team of equal ability.

- Games should last 8 minutes.

- Rules for half-court basketball apply; ball needs to be brought back to the center line after a team scores.

- Teachers should not coach students during game play.

- Students should call their own out-of-bounds and rules violations, and keep score.

- Start and stop the camera and game at the same time. If using two cameras, you can run two games at the same time.

Safety:

- Make sure that courts are free from obstruction.

Equipment/Materials:

- Regulation-size boys basketballs.

- Numbered pinnies of different colors for offense and defense.

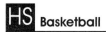

Diagram of Space/Distances:

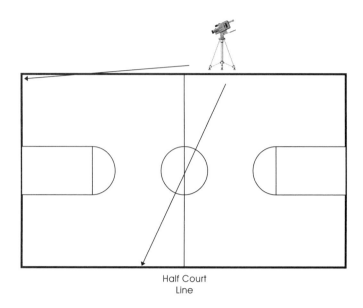

Half Court
Line

Camera Location/Operation:

The camera should be placed as shown, with the zoom open wide so the circle at center court is at the bottom edge of the screen and the back line of the court is at the top of the screen. Once a game starts, the camera can be left on in the above position until the game is over.

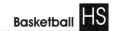

Assessment Score Sheet

PE Teacher _____   Grade _____   Date _____

School _____   Classroom Teacher _____

Pinnie Number	Student Name	Gender	Grade	Ball Skills (0-4)	Offensive Play (0-4)	Individual Defensive Play (0-4)	Team Defense (0-4)	Total Score (0-16) 12=Competent

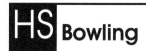 Bowling

Note: This is a useful assessment. However, because of a small sample size, the ability score for this assessment cannot be calculated.

Standard 1:

Demonstrates competency in motor skills and movement patterns needed to perform a variety of physical activities.

Performance Indicator:

Demonstrate competence in individual/dual competitive activities.

Assessment Task:

Bowl and score 10 frames, using an appropriate-weight ball.

Criteria for Competence (Level 3):

1. Demonstrates 3 essential elements for set-up and delivery on both trials:

    a) Begins with shoulders square to lane and in a still position.

    b) Uses 4- or 5-step approach, including opposition on release.

    c) Executes smooth delivery, with backswing and follow-through (pendulum swing).

    d) Releases ball low to ground.

2. Bowls a score between 80 and 99 in 10 frames.

3. Scores 10 frames with no more than 1 error.

■ Assessment Rubric:

Level	1. Set-Up & Delivery	2. Total Bowling Score	3. Scoring
4	Demonstrates all 4 essential elements on both trials.	Bowls a score of 100 or above.	Scores 10 frames with no errors.
3	Demonstrates 3 essential elements for set-up and delivery on both trials: a. Begins with shoulders square to lane and in a still position. b. Uses 4- or 5-step approach, including opposition on release. c. Executes smooth delivery, with backswing and follow-through (pendulum swing), d. Releases ball low to ground.	Bowls a score between 80 and 99 in 10 frames.	Scores 10 frames with no more than 1 error.
2	Demonstrates 2 of 4 essential elements on both trials.	Bowls a score between 60 and 79.	Scores 10 frames with no more than 2 errors.
1	Demonstrates 1 or none of the essential elements.	Bowls a score of 59 or below.	Scores 10 frames with 3 or more errors.
0	Violates safety procedures and/or does not complete the assessment task.		

■ Assessment Protocols:

Directions for Students (Read aloud, verbatim):

- You will be asked to bowl 10 frames.

- You will be assessed on:

  a) Having your shoulders square to lane and in a still position.

  b) Using a 4- or 5-step approach, including opposition on release.

  c) Executing a smooth delivery, with backswing and follow-through.

  d) Releasing the ball low to the ground.

  e) Your ability to keep score.

  f) You also will be evaluated on your total score.

Directions for Teachers:

Preparation:

- See the chapter titled Administering & Scoring PE Metrics Assessments for instruction and warm-up.

- The testing should occur at a regulation bowling facility.

- If electronic scoring is available, it should be turned off.

- Students can be tested in groups of 4 (possibly 5 or 6) in two adjacent lanes that are served by the same ball-return.

- Although students will be assessed on their ability to score and their total bowling score for 10 frames, they will be assessed on their set-up and approach for only 2 frames. Therefore, after filming students on adjacent lanes for 2 frames, rotate new students to the lanes being filmed. Continue this procedure until all students are filmed.

- Provide students with scoring sheets and pencils. Students will perform their own scoring. Score sheets should be turned in to the teacher.

- Students should be permitted to bowl two warm-up balls prior to scoring.

- For safety purposes, and to improve camera viewability, students should not be permitted to stand behind a bowler.

Safety:

- Students should use the appropriate ball and shoes.

- The lanes should be free from liquids or materials that would be dangerous.

Equipment/Materials:

- Regulation bowling alley.

- Large-enough selection of balls and shoes so that every student is equipped appropriately.

- Numbered pinnies.

Diagram of Space/Distances:

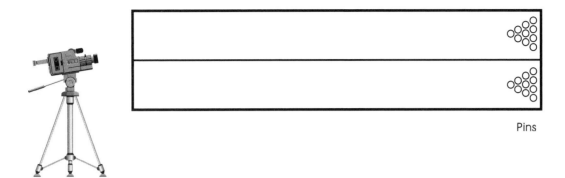

Pins

Camera Location/Operation:

Camera should be placed in back of two inside lanes. Both lanes should be visible in the camera view so that students' entire bodies and their approaches can be seen. The camera can run without being turned off during the 2 frames being assessed.

Assessment Score Sheet

PE Teacher _____   Grade _____   Date _____

School _____   Classroom Teacher _____

Pinnie Number	Student Name	Gender	Grade	Setup and Delivery (0-4)	Total Bowling Score (0-4)	Scoring (0-4)	Total Score (0-12) 9=Competent

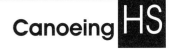

Standard 1:

Demonstrates competency in motor skills and movement patterns needed to perform a variety of physical activities.

Performance Indicator:

Demonstrate competency in adventure/outdoor activities.

Assessment Task:

Paddle a canoe through a 25-yard course.

Criteria for Competence (Level 3):

1. Enters and exits canoe using appropriate techniques and safety procedures, with no more than one error.

2. Paddles canoe in straight line, with no more than 1 deviation in each direction in bow and stern position and on each side.

3. Makes U-turn around buoy, staying within 6 feet of the buoy.

4. Demonstrates 3 of the 4 essential elements for good technique:

   a). Proper grip.

   b). Entry phase (proper angle of paddle at entry).

   c). Power phase (blade perpendicular to the direction of the pull).

   d). Recovery phase (proper feathering in or out of the water).

5. Usually coordinates efforts with partner to complete the course.

■ **Assessment Rubric:**

Level	1. Entry, Exit, Safety	2. Paddles Canoe in Straight Line	3. U-Turn	4. Stroke Technique	5. Coordination With Partner
4	Enters and exits canoe using appropriate techniques and safety procedures* with no errors.	Paddles canoe in straight line, with no deviation in both bow and stern position and on each side.	Makes a smooth, tight U-turn around buoy, without touching the buoy.	Demonstrates all essential elements for good technique.	Consistently coordinates efforts with partner to complete the course smoothly.
3	Enters and exits canoe using appropriate techniques and safety procedures, with no more than 1 error.	Paddles canoe in straight line, with no more than 1 deviation in each direction in bow and stern position and on each side.	Makes U-turn around buoy, staying within 6 feet of the buoy.	Demonstrates 3 of the 4 essential elements for good technique: a) proper grip; b) entry phase (proper angle of paddle at entry); c) power phase (blade perpendicular to the direction of the pull); d) recovery phase (proper feathering in or out of the water).	Usually coordinates efforts with partner to complete the course.
2	Enters and exits canoe using appropriate techniques, with no more than 2 errors.	Paddles canoe in straight line, with no more than 2 deviations in each direction in bow and stern position and on each side.	Makes wide U-turn around buoy, moving away from the buoy more than 6 feet, or hits the buoy.	Demonstrates 2 of the 4 essential elements for good technique.	Sometimes coordinates efforts with partner to complete the course.
1	Enters and exits canoe using appropriate techniques, with more than 2 errors.	Paddles canoe in straight line, with no more than 3 deviations in each direction in bow and stern positions and on each side.	Unable to make U-turn around buoy.	Demonstrates 1 or none of essential elements for good technique.	Seldom coordinates efforts with partner to complete the course or fails to complete at least one of the components .
0	Violates safety procedures and/or does not complete the assessment task.				

* Safety techniques: Enter: anchor canoe, place hand on gunwale, place foot in center and reach to far gunwale to balance weight. Keep weight low and centered in canoe. Reverse procedure to exit.

Scoring: Consistently = 90% or above; Usually = 75% – 89%; Sometimes = 50% – 74%; Seldom = below 50%

■ **Assessment Protocols:**

Directions for Students (Read aloud, verbatim):

- You will be asked to enter and paddle a canoe on a straight course, to the buoy, with the stern paddler paddling on the side closest to the camera.

- Turn at a buoy 25 yards away, using a U-turn around the buoy.

- Change the side that you are paddling on and return to the starting point.

- Exit the canoe, change bow and stern positions, and repeat.

- You will be assessed on your ability to:
    - a)   Use appropriate techniques to enter and exit the canoe.
    - b)   Follow safety procedures.
    - c)   Choose the appropriate strokes to paddle a straight course in both positions and on both sides.
    - d)   Choose the appropriate strokes to make a tight U-turn in both positions.
    - e)   Use proper stroke technique.
    - f)   Coordinate efforts with your partner to complete the task.

Directions for Teachers:
Preparations:

- See the chapter titled Administering & Scoring PE Metrics Assessments for instruction and warm-up.

- Lay out a course with a buoy 25 yards from the entry point, in calm water or in a swimming pool at least 25 yards long.

- Arrange students in partners of equal ability. Students should have mastered the following strokes before attempting this task: bow, back, J-stroke, forward and reverse sweeps, draw, push-over (pry).

- You can test two canoes at a time, provided that the first canoe reaches the turn before the second canoe starts the course (lake only).

- Have students enter the canoe, begin and end, and exit the canoe at the start/finish line.

- Allow students to choose which stroke(s) to use for each component.

Safety:

- All students should follow safety regulations of canoeing.

- All students should wear a life preserver.

- More than one adult should be in the assessment area.

- At least one adult should be a certified lifeguard.

Equipment/Materials:

- Life preserver of appropriate size for each student.

- A canoe and paddles (of appropriate size).

- A buoy, placed 25 yards from the starting point.

- Numbered pinnies.

Diagram of Space/Distances:

Lake:

- - - = Path of Canoe

○ = Buoy

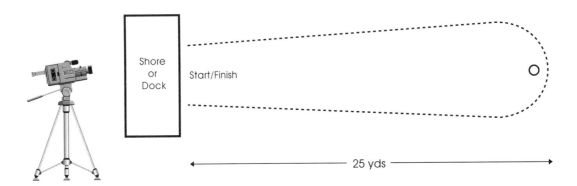

POOL : Set the course at a diagonal, with enough space to make the turn at the buoy, which should be set at least 9 feet from the end or side of the pool.

Camera Location/Operation:

Plsace the camera 20 feet behind the point at which students will enter the canoe. You can leave it running unattended while students are being tested if you can see the buoy from that point. Take care that glare from the water does not interfere with the picture.

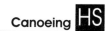

Assessment Score Sheet

PE Teacher _____ Grade _____ Date _____

School _____ Classroom Teacher _____

Pinnie Number	Student Name	Gender	Grade	Safety (0-4)	Pathway				U-Turn		Stroke Technique		Coordination With Partner	Total Score (0-40) 30=Competent
					Bow (0-8)		Stern (0-8)		Bow (0-4)	Stern (0-4)	Bow (0-4)	Stern (0-4)	Stern (0-4)	
					P	S	P	S						

HS Flag Football

Note: This is a useful assessment. However, because of a small sample size, the ability score for this assessment might not be accurate.

Standard 1:

Demonstrates competency in motor skills and movement patterns needed to perform a variety of physical activities.

Performance Indicator:

Demonstrate competence in team field sports.

Assessment Task:

Play a modified game of 3-on-3 flag football with a quarterback and two pass receivers on each team.

Criteria for Competence (Level 3):

1. Throws 2 catchable passes.
2. Usually runs a recognizable pattern.
3. Usually catches catchable passes.
4. Consistently positions self to intercept the ball.

■ Assessment Rubric:

Level	1. Quarterback	2. Receiver Patterns	3. Receiver Catches	4. Defensive Player
4	Throws 3 catchable passes.	Consistently runs a recognizable pattern that eludes defenders.	Consistently catches catchable passes.	Always positions self to intercept the ball.
3	Throws 2 catchable passes.	Usually runs a recognizable pattern.	Usually catches catchable passes.	Consistently positions self to intercept the ball.
2	Throws 1 catchable pass.	Sometimes runs a recognizable pattern.	Sometimes catches catchable passes.	Usually positions self to intercept the ball.
1	Throws no catchable passes.	Seldom runs a recognizable pattern.	Seldom catches catchable passes.	Sometimes or seldom positions self to intercept the ball.
0	Violates safety procedures and/or does not complete the assessment task.			

Scoring: Always = 100%; Consistently = 90% – 99%; Usually = 75% – 89%; Sometimes or Seldom = below 75%

■ Assessment Protocols:

Directions for Students (Read aloud, verbatim):

- You will be asked to play a modified game of flag football on a short and narrow field.

- There will be no blocking or tackling.

- There will be 3 players on each team. The offense must huddle to call a pass pattern for each receiver.

- On offense, each team will complete 9 plays.

- On defense, the team will attempt to stop the offense for 9 plays. Each defender will play person-on-person defense.

- The offense will begin play on the start line and run 9 consecutive plays, rotating quarterbacks every 3 passes. Each player will play quarterback for 3 plays.

- Only the quarterback will wear a flag.

- One defender must rush the quarterback *after* a 3-second count.

- Each quarterback must pass on each play.

- If the offense loses possession of the ball due to interception, incomplete pass, ball batted away or the defense pulls the quarterback's flag before the pass is made, the offense begins a new play until its 9 passes are complete.

- Each receiver must have an opportunity to receive catchable passes. If each receiver does not have 3 opportunities to catch the ball, play will continue.

- You will be assessed on your ability to:
    - a) Throw catchable passes.
    - b) Run a recognizable pattern.
    - c) Catch catchable passes.
    - d) Position yourself to intercept the ball when defending.

Directions for Teachers:
Preparation:

- See the chapter titled Administering & Scoring PE Metrics Assessments for instruction and warm-up.

- Teams of similar skill ability should be determined prior to the assessment.

- The offensive team takes possession of the ball at the start line.

- All plays begin at the start line.

- Following each pass play, the ball is returned to the start line.

- The snap occurs when the ball is picked up from the start line.

- If, after rotating through the assessment, not all students have had an opportunity to receive 3 passes, select a quarterback and tell students to continue playing until each has had 3 opportunities to receive the ball. The quarter back and defenders will not be assessed again during these extra plays. Only the receiver will be assessed.

Safety:

- Make sure that the field is clear of all obstructions.

- Enforce all rules, without exception, to maintain safe play.

Equipment/Materials:

- Numbered pinnies of different colors for offense and defense.

- One flag belt for the quarterback.

- Intermediate-size football.

- A line of scrimmage (10 yards into playing area), marked by cones as a start-of-play marker.

- Outdoor field area.

Diagram of Space/Distances:

Field is 40 yards long (width of a regulation football field) and 30 yards wide (one-third of the length of a regulation football field).

△ = Cone (marks line of scrimmage)

Q = Quarterback

O = Offensive Receiver

D = Defensive Player

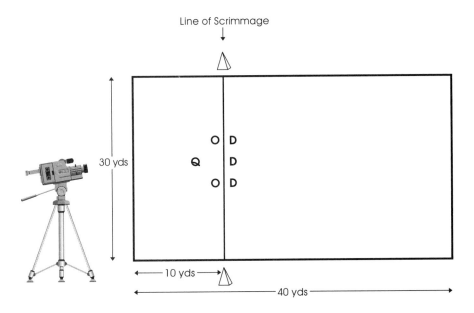

Camera Location/Operation:

Play should be filmed from behind the Quarterback start line. The camera should be close enough so that all players are in view for the entire assessment. The lens angle should be adjusted wide enough to include the movements of all players from both teams in the viewfinder. The camera should follow the action of all players involved on the team. Camera movement to follow players should be smooth. If including all players is not possible, at least be sure to include the ball-handler in the viewfinder. The camera should be left running during the assessment.

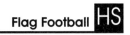

Assessment Score Sheet

PE Teacher _____   Grade _____   Date _____

School _____   Classroom Teacher _____

Pinnie Number	Student Name	Gender	Grade	Quarterback (0-4)	Receiver Patterns (0-4)	Receiver Catches (0-4)	Defensive Player (0-4)	Total Score (0-16) 12=Competent

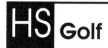

HS Golf

Standard 1:

Demonstrates competency in motor skills and movement patterns needed to perform a variety of physical activities.

Performance Indicator:

Demonstrate competency in individual/dual competitive sports.

Assessment Task:

Demonstrate a pre-swing stance and full swing in golf.

Criteria for Competence (Level 3):

1. Demonstrates 5 of the 7 essential elements of appropriate pre-swing stance for full swing (grip, set-up).

2. Displays 5 of the 7 essential elements of a full swing for the best of 3 trials.

3. Ball trajectory is appropriate for club selected for the full swing for 2 of the 3 trials.

■ Assessment Rubric:

Level	1. Pre-Swing	2. Full Swing	3. Ball Trajectory
4	Demonstrates 6 or 7 of the essential elements of appropriate pre-swing stance for full swing (grip, set-up).	Displays 6 or 7 of the essential elements of a full swing for the best of 3 trials.	Ball trajectory is appropriate for club selected for full swing for all 3 trials.
3	Demonstrates 5 of the 7 essential elements of appropriate pre-swing stance for full swing (grip, set-up).	Displays 5 of the 7 essential elements of a full swing for the best of 3 trials.	Ball trajectory is appropriate for club selected for full swing for 2 of the 3 trials.
2	Demonstrates 3 or 4 of the essential elements of appropriate pre-swing stance for full swing (grip, set-up).	Displays 3 or 4 of the essential elements of a full swing for the best of 3 trials.	Ball trajectory is appropriate for club selected for full swing for 1 of the 3 trials.
1	Demonstrates fewer than 3 of the essential elements of appropriate pre-swing stance for full swing (grip, set-up).	Displays fewer than 3 of the essential elements of a full swing for the best of 3 trials.	Ball trajectory is not appropriate for club selected for full swing for any of the 3 trials.
0	Violates safety procedures and/or does not complete the assessment task.		

■ **Essential Elements:**

1. Pre-Swing (7 points maximum):

   A. Grip:

      1. Uses overlap, interlocking or 10-finger grip.

      2. Club more in fingers than palm.

      3. Hands in neutral position.

   B. Set-Up:

      1. Feet approximately shoulder-width apart.

      2. Knees bent slightly.

      3. Hands even or slightly ahead of ball.

      4. Ball position between center and inside front heel.

2. Full Swing (7 points maximum):

    1. Displays rotational motion.

    2. Left arm (for right-handed golfers) extended or just slightly flexed at top of backswing.

    3. Club parallel or just short of parallel to ground at top of backswing.

    4. Head stays relatively level throughout backswing to impact.

    5. Club swings through the ball to finish position over target-side shoulder.

    6. Belt buckle finishes facing target.

    7. Weight transferred to target-side foot at completion of swing.

3. Trajectory (acceptable or not acceptable)

Trajectory (loft of ball) is appropriate for club selected for full swing.

■ **Assessment Protocols:**

Directions for Students (Read aloud, verbatim):

- You will be asked to demonstrate a pre-swing stance, a full swing, a chip shot and a putt.

- You will hit three balls for each shot.

- You will be given 5 minutes to warm up using each shot before you are assessed.

- Choose an iron, with which you hit a ball less than 100 yards, to demonstrate a shot with a full swing.

1. Pre-Swing Stance

- You will be assessed on:

a) Grip.

- Overlap, interlocking, or 10-finger grip.
- Club more in fingers than palm.
- Hands in neutral position.

b) Set-Up.

- Feet approximately shoulder-width apart.
- Knees bent slightly.
- Hands even or slightly ahead of ball.
- Ball position between center and inside front heel.

2. Full Swing

- You will be assessed on:

a) Rotation.

b) Left arm position.

c) Club position at the top and end of your swing.

d) Your head remaining level.

e) Club following through to finish position.

f) Body finishing facing the target.

g) Weight shifting to the front foot.

3. Trajectory

- You will be assessed on the height of the ball. The ball should rise to 20 or 30 feet in height, or about the height of a 2-story building.

Directions for Teachers:

Preparation:

- See the chapter titled Administering & Scoring PE Metrics Assessments for instruction and warm-up.

- Assign students their order for testing. Assign all left-handed players at one time, as you will have to move the camera for them.

- Allow all students to warm up with whatever clubs (no balls) they wish for 5 minutes.

- For the full swing (no tee), have the student face the camera and take his/her grip while holding the club upright and then in a normal starting position. Zoom in on the grip. When finished filming the grip, give the student a signal that he/she can line up to hit the first ball. Video the student hitting the ball 3 times. **Important:** Because it will not be possible for the camera to record the trajectory of the ball in the full swing, the teacher should state whether the trajectory of the ball is "acceptable" or "not acceptable" after each trial so that the microphone on the camera can record the statement. To be "acceptable," the ball should rise to 20 or 30 feet in height, or about the height of a 2-story building.

- Teachers should not coach students.

Safety:

- Do not allow students to swing any club close to another student.

- Do not allow students to recover balls until everyone has finished taking his/her shots.

- Do not allow students to walk behind students who are swinging a club.

- Be sure that students do not choose a club for the full swing that will help them hit the ball farther than the distance you have available.

Equipment:

- Clubs: 5 iron to pitching wedge for the full swing (enough for the number of students practicing and being assessed at one time).

- Space: Outdoor field at least 100 yards long, with a target (cone, flag) at the end of the field.

- Numbered pinnies.

Diagram of Space/Distances:

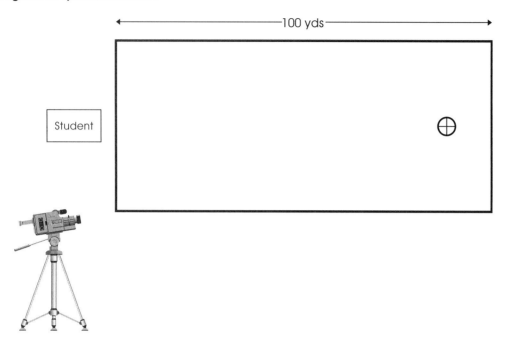

←————————————————100 yds————————————————→

Student

Camera Location/Operation:

For the full swing, the camera should be placed to the side of the "start" line. Each student should move to position at the "start" line. The student should take the set-up position, the camera should zoom in and focus on the grip, then zoom back so that the whole student is visible for the full swing.

Assessment Score Sheet

PE Teacher _____   Grade _____   Date _____

School _____   Classroom Teacher _____

Pinnie Number	Student Name	Gender	Grade	Pre-Swing (0-4)	Full Swing (0-4) Best of 3 Trials	Ball Trajectory (0-4)	Total Score (0-12) 9= Competence

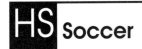 Soccer

Standard 1:

Demonstrates competency in motor skills and movement patterns needed to perform a variety of physical activities.

Performance Indicator:

Demonstrate competence in team field sports.

Assessment Task:

Play a modified game of 3-on-3 soccer.

Criteria for Competence (Level 3):

1. Usually demonstrates good ball control (dribbling, passing, trapping/receiving, shooting).
2. Usually demonstrates good offensive play (moves to open space to receive a pass and uses effective lead passes).
3. Usually demonstrates good defensive play (maintains good defensive position against an opponent and tackles with good body control).

■ Assessment Rubric:

Level	1. Ball Control	2. Offensive Techniques	3. Defensive Techniques
4	Consistently demonstrates good ball control.	Consistently demonstrates good offensive play.	Consistently demonstrates good defensive play.
3	Usually demonstrates good ball control (dribbling, passing, trapping/receiving, shooting).	Usually demonstrates good offensive play (moves to open space to receive a pass and uses effective lead passes).	Usually demonstrates good defensive play (maintains good defensive position against an opponent and tackles with good body control).
2	Sometimes demonstrates good ball control.	Sometimes demonstrates good offensive play.	Sometimes demonstrates good defensive play.
1	Seldom demonstrates good ball control.	Seldom demonstrates good offensive play.	Seldom demonstrates good defensive play.
0	Violates safety procedures and/or does not complete the assessment task.		

Scoring: Consistently = 90% or above; Usually = 75% – 89% ; Sometimes = 50% – 74%; Seldom = below 50%

■ Assessment Protocols:

Directions for Students (Read aloud, verbatim):

- You will play a modified game of soccer with 3 people on a side, no goalkeeper, for 6 minutes.

- Change sides of field after 3 minutes.

- The 3 people on your team can choose the positions they want to play.

- You may switch positions during game play, if you want.

- You will be expected to apply the rules of the game and engage in safe and legal play.

- You will be assessed on:

    1) Good ball control (dribbling, passing, trapping/receiving, shooting).

    2) Good offensive play (moves to open space to receive a pass and uses effective lead passes).

    3) Good defensive play (maintains good defensive position against an opponent and tackles with good body control).

- For a goal to count, it must pass through the goal area without hitting the cone.

Directions for Teachers:
Preparation:

- See the chapter titled Administering & Scoring PE Metrics Assessments for instruction and warm-up.

- Assign students to be tested to two teams of 3 players that are matched by ability.

Safety:

- Be sure that the field is free of all obstacles.

Equipment/Materials:

- Four regulation-size 5 soccer balls.

- A modified and marked 40- x 30-yard outdoor playing field is needed, with two goals (or half a soccer field).

- Two 24-inch cones, placed 5 feet apart, should mark the goal.

- Numbered pinnies of different colors for offense and defense.

Diagram of Space/Distances:

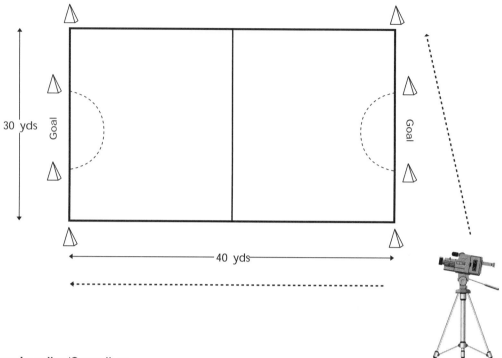

Camera Location/Operation:

Play should be filmed from the back corner of the field. The camera should be elevated with a wide-angle view, so that most of the playing field is in view at all times. Start the camera prior to starting the game, and stop it after the game ends. All player numbers must be identifiable.

Assessment Score Sheet

PE Teacher _____   Grade _____   Date _____

School _____   Classroom Teacher _____

Pinnie Number	Student Name	Gender	Grade	Ball Control (0-4)	Offensive Techniques (0-4)	Defensive Techniques (0-4)	Total Score (0-12) 9=Competent

HS Swimming

Standard 1:

Demonstrates competency in motor skills and movement patterns needed to perform a variety of physical activities.

Performance Indicator:

Demonstrate competency in individual/non-competitive sports.

Assessment Task:

Swim in both prone (face-down) and supine (face-up) positions and tread water.

Criteria for Competence (Level 3):

1. Can swim a distance of 25 yards in a prone position, without stopping, using the same stroke.
2. Can swim a distance of 25 yards in a supine position, without stopping, using the same stroke.
3. Can tread water for 1 minute without undue stress. (May use more than one strategy.)

■ Assessment Rubric:

Level	1. Swim Prone	2. Swim Supine	3. Tread Water
4	Swims a distance of 25 yards in a prone position effortlessly, using the same stroke.	Swims a distance of 25 yards in a supine position effortlessly, using the same stroke.	Treads water effortlessly for 1 minute.
3	Swims a distance of 25 yards in a prone position, without stopping, using the same stroke.	Swims a distance of 25 yards in a supine position, without stopping, using the same stroke.	Treads water for 1 minute without undue stress. (May use more than one strategy.)
2	Completes the 25 yards but struggles and/or uses more than one stroke.	Completes the 25 yards but struggles and/or uses more than one stroke.	Struggles to tread water for 1 minute.
1	Does not swim 25 yards or must stop and then continue.	Does not swim 25 yards or must stop and then continue.	Does not complete 1 minute without going under or touching the side of the pool.
0	Violates safety procedures and/or does not complete the assessment task.		

■ **Assessment Protocols:**

Directions for Students (Read aloud, verbatim):

- You will be asked to swim 25 yards in the prone (face-down) position and 25 yards in the supine (face-up) position continuously.

- You are not being assessed on speed.

- You may use any single stroke for the face-up position and any single stroke for the face-down position.

- You also will be asked to tread water for a period of 1 minute without stopping.

- You will be assessed on your ability to:
  a) Swim the distance face up using one single stroke and face down using one single stroke.
  b) Tread water for 1 minute without going under.

Directions for Teachers:
Preparation:

- See the chapter titled Administering & Scoring PE Metrics Assessments for instruction and warm-up.

- The camera must see each student (with a number) out of the water before he/she swims. (Place numbers on pool deck by lanes in which individual students are swimming so that they are visible to the camera.)

- You may test more than 1 student at a time, depending on camera angle and whether a lifeguard is present. Usually, 3 or 4 students can swim at one time.

- Students should swim 25 yards, without stopping, in either supine or prone position. They may rest before beginning the next 25 yards. You may have every student do one part of the test before beginning the second/third part.

- Assess treading water in groups of 3 students. Ensure that students are close enough to the camera for viewer to see them.

Safety:

- A lifeguard should be present for large classes.

- Teachers should have water safety instructor certifications or the equivalent.

- Students who present a safety hazard to themselves or others should not be assessed.

- All safety regulations for teaching swimming should apply.

Equipment/Materials:

- A stopwatch, numbers and a way to signal students when time is up.

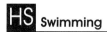
Diagram of Space/Distances:

The ideal facility is a pool 25 yards long. If that's not available, allow students to turn at a wall (without stopping or touching the bottom). Place markers to designate when 25 yards is completed from the starting line.

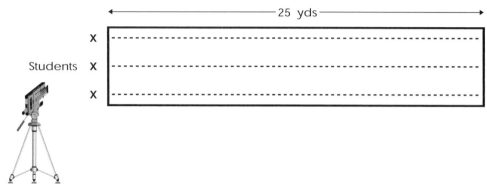

Camera Location/Operation:

Place the camera facing the starting line, at a point where you can see students — and their numbers — during the entire assessment. This is likely to be different for each pool set-up.

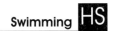

Assessment Score Sheet

PE Teacher _____ Grade _____ Date _____

School _____ Classroom Teacher _____

Pinnie Number	Student Name	Gender	Grade	Swim Prone (0-4)	Swim Supine (0-4)	Treads Water (0-4)	Total Score (0-12) 9=Competent

HS Tennis

Note: This is a useful assessment. However, because of a small sample size, the ability score for this assessment cannot be calculated.

Standard 1:

Demonstrates competency in motor skills and movement patterns needed to perform a variety of physical activities.

Performance Indicator:

Demonstrate competence in individual/dual sports.

Assessment Task:

Play 2 games or 6 minutes of tennis singles, whichever comes first.

Criteria for Competence (Level 3):

1. Usually puts the ball into play using a legal overhand serve.
2. Usually uses a technically correct forehand or backhand ground stroke (racket preparation, turn to side, contact point, follow-through).
3. Usually chooses to use the forehand or backhand ground stroke appropriately.
4. Usually attempts to hit into open space away from the opponent.
5. Usually returns a playable ball over the net into opposing court.
6. Usually follows rules and etiquette, keeps score and calls out-of-bounds balls correctly.

■ Assessment Rubric:

Level	1. Serve	2. Ground Strokes	3. Choice of Strokes	4. Hits to Open Spaces	5. Returns Ball	6. Rules
4	Consistently puts the ball into play using a legal overhand serve.	Consistently uses a technically correct ground stroke (forehand or backhand).	Consistently chooses to use the forehand or backhand ground stroke appropriately.	Consistently attempts to hit into open space, away from the opponent.	Consistently returns a playable* ball over the net, into opposing court.	Consistently follows rules and etiquette, keeps score and calls out-of-bounds balls correctly.
3	Usually puts the ball into play using a legal overhand serve.	Usually uses a technically correct forehand or backhand ground stroke (racquet preparation; turn to side; contact point; follow-through).	Usually chooses to use the forehand or backhand ground stroke appropriately.	Usually attempts to hit into open space, away from the opponent.	Usually returns a playable* ball over the net, into opposing court.	Usually follows rules and etiquette, keeps score and calls out-of-bounds balls correctly.
2	Sometimes puts the ball into play using a legal overhand serve.	Sometimes uses a technically correct ground stroke (forehand or backhand).	Sometimes chooses to use the forehand or backhand ground stroke appropriately.	Sometimes attempts to hit into open space, away from the opponent.	Sometimes returns a playable* ball over the net, into opposing court.	Sometimes follows rules and etiquette, keeps score and calls out-of-bounds balls correctly.
1	Seldom is able to put the ball into play; hits into the net or outside the service area.	Seldom uses a technically correct ground stroke (forehand or backhand).	Seldom chooses to use the forehand or backhand ground stroke appropriately.	Seldom attempts to hit into open space, away from the opponent.	Seldom returns a playable* ball over the net, into opposing court.	Seldom follows rules and etiquette, keeps score and calls out-of-bounds balls correctly.
0	Violates safety procedures and/or does not complete the assessment task.					

*A playable ball is one that a player should reasonably be able to reach.

Scoring: Consistently = above 90%; Usually = 75% – 89%; Sometimes = 50% – 74%; Seldom = below 50%

■ Assessment Protocols:

Directions for Students (Read aloud, verbatim):

- You will be asked to play two games or 6 minutes of singles tennis, whichever comes first.

- Each player will serve one game.

- Both servers will serve from the court nearest the camera, so players will change sides after game 1.

- The person serving will call out the score before serving.

- No one game will be more than 3 minutes.

- You will be assessed on your ability to:
  - Put the ball into play using a legal overhand serve.
  - Use a technically correct forehand or backhand ground stroke (racquet preparation, turn to side, contact point, follow-through).
  - Choose a forehand or a backhand ground stroke, when appropriate.
  - Attempt to hit into open space, away from the opponent.
  - Return a playable ball over the net, into the opposing court.
  - Follow rules and etiquette, keep score and call out-of-bounds balls correctly.

Directions for Teachers:

Preparation:

- See the chapter titled Administering & Scoring PE Metrics Assessments for instruction and warm-up.

- Students should be paired with others of similar ability.

- Allow up to 3 minutes for each game.

- Provide a ball retriever for each court, if possible, to speed up the game, and place ball retrievers well behind the baselines.

Safety:

- Clear the courts of any obstacles or water.

- No students should be on the courts while play is in progress, except the ball retrievers.

- Check rackets prior to play; do not use rackets with handle cracks or broken strings.

- Loose tennis balls should be removed from the playing area.

- Instruct retrievers to be sure that players are looking at them before tossing balls back.

Equipment/Materials:

- Two regulation courts are preferable, so that 4 students can be assessed at one time.

- A racket for each player.

- Two tennis balls for each player.

Diagram of Space/Distances:

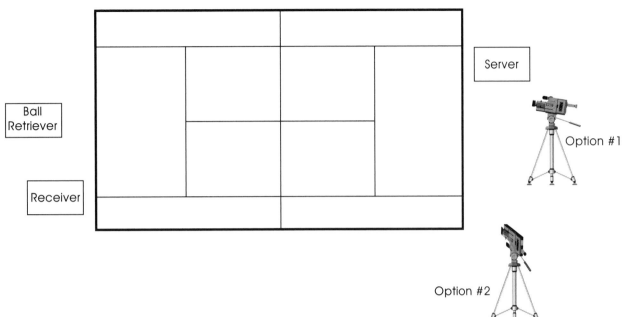

Camera Location/Operation:

The assessment will require one camcorder for each court. Place the camera far enough away so as to view both sides of court with as large a picture as possible. Keep the camera stationary and recording, once play has started. Keep the sound on. Each game should be recorded in full.

If two cameras are available, set up an identical assessment situations and assess 4 students at a time.

If space is adequate behind the court, center the camera at that location. If not, place camera at corner of court.

Assessment Score Sheet

PE Teacher _____   Grade _____   Date _____

School _____   Classroom Teacher _____

Pinnie Number	Student Name	Gender	Grade	Serve (0-4)	Ground Strokes (0-4)	Choice of Strokes (0-4)	Hits to Open Spaces (0-4)	Returns Ball (0-4)	Rules (0-4)	Total Score (0-24) 18=Competent

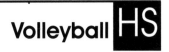
Standard 1:

Demonstrates competency in motor skills and movement patterns needed to perform a variety of physical activities.

Performance Indicator:

Demonstrate competency in team court sports.

Assessment Task:

Play a modified game of 4-v.-4 volleyball.

Criteria for Competence (Level 3):

1. Usually sends a playable forearm pass to a teammate or over the net with good technique.
2. Usually sends a playable overhead pass to a teammate or over the net with good technique.
3. Usually puts the ball in play with a legal serve.

■ Assessment Rubric:

Level	1. Forearm Passing Technique	2. Overhead Passing Technique	3. Serve
4	Consistently sends a playable* forearm pass to a teammate or over the net with good technique.	Consistently sends a playable* overhead pass to a teammate or over the net with good technique.	Consistently puts the ball in play with a legal serve, sometimes difficult to return (e.g., spin, placement, form).
3	Usually sends a playable forearm pass to a teammate or over the net with good technique.	Usually sends a playable overhead pass to a teammate or over the net with good technique.	Usually puts the ball in play with a legal serve.
2	Sometimes sends a playable forearm pass to a teammate or over the net with good technique.	Sometimes sends a playable overhead pass to a teammate or over the net with good technique.	Sometimes puts the ball in play with a legal serve.
1	Seldom sends a playable forearm pass to a teammate or over the net with good technique.	Seldom sends a playable overhead pass to a teammate or over the net with good technique.	Seldom puts the ball in play with a legal serve.
0	Violates safety procedures and/or does not complete the assessment task.		

*A playable ball is one that a player should reasonably be able to reach.

Scoring: Consistently = 90% or above; Usually = 75% – 89%; Sometimes = 50% – 74%; Seldom = below 50%

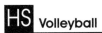

■ Assessment Protocols:

Directions for Students (Read aloud, verbatim):

- You will be asked to play a modified game of volleyball with 4 people on a side, for at least 20 minutes, or as long as needed to allow every player on the court to serve at least 4 times, alternating service after every point.

- Change sides of court after 10 minutes.

- You will be assessed on your ability to use the forearm pass, overhead pass and serve from behind the service line, with good technique.

- All the rules of volleyball will be used, except that you will:
    a) Alternate serves with the other team, regardless of who scores.
    b) Call out your number just prior to serving the ball.
    c) Play on a modified-size court that has been identified by boundary markings on the floor.

Directions for Teachers:
Preparation:

- See the chapter titled Administering & Scoring PE Metrics Assessments for instruction and warm-up.

- Assign students to teams of 4 students, in a manner that would best allow students to display their ability.

- Assign teams to play each other.

- Start each game and the camera at the same time.

- For scoring purposes, focus only on the serve, forearm pass and underhand pass and not on other responses (e.g., spike, dink, dig).

Safety:

- Floor is to be dry, clean and clear of obstacles at least beyond the boundary of the court.

Equipment/Materials:

- Regulation leather vollyeballs.

- Clearly mark a 20' x 40- volleyball court. Net should be 7 feet, 6 inches high. Mark the net with tape or string to indicate the 20' boundary.

- Numbered pinnies.

Diagram of Space/Distances:

X = Player
S = Server

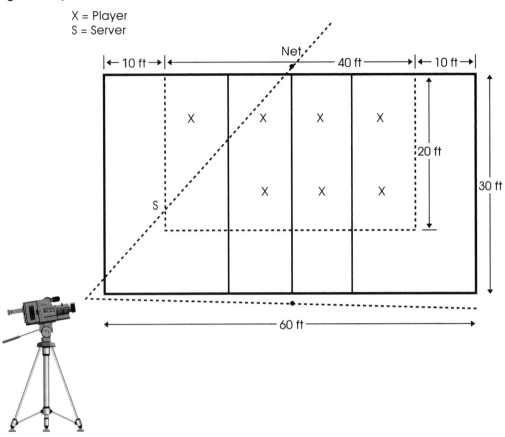

Camera Location/Operation:

You have two options for camera placement, depending upon the gym's configuration:

One option is to place the camera high to be able to see both sides of one whole court clearly. If it is difficult to find a camera placement high enough to allow a full view of the whole court and all players, set the camera as high as possible and at an angle to the right of the serving position to allow a view of the right part of the forecourt and a good view of the entire other court. When the teams exchange sides after 10 minutes, the camera should remain where it is. Keep the camera stationary and recording once play has started. Each game should be recorded for at least 20 minutes, and at least 4 serves by every player, with an exchange of sides after 10 minutes.

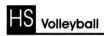

Assessment Score Sheet

PE Teacher _____ Grade _____ Date _____

School _____ Classroom Teacher _____

Pinnie Number	Student Name	Gender	Grade	Forearm Passing Technique (0-4)	Overhead Passing Technique (0-4)	Serve (0-4)	Total Score (0-12) 9=Competent

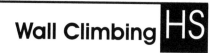
Note: This is a useful assessment. However, because of a small sample size, the ability score for this assessment might not be accurate.

Standard 1:

Demonstrates competency in motor skills and movement patterns needed to perform a variety of physical activities

Performance Indicator:

Demonstrate competence in adventure/outdoor activities

Assessment Task:

Climb a vertical wall.

Criteria for Competence (Level 3):

1. Usually demonstrates essential elements for good technique:

    a) Maintains 3 points of contact.

    b) Uses proper foot position.

    c) Keeps hips close to wall.

    d) Uses legs to support weight and uses handholds for balance.

2. Usually executes well-planned movements, with few observable realignments.

3. Climbs at a smooth, steady pace, with some hesitation, to the top.

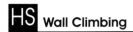

■ **Assessment Rubric:**

Level	1. Technique	2. Body Efficiency	3. Complete Climb
4	Consistently demonstrates essential elements for good technique.	Consistently executes well-planned movements, with smooth, efficient transitions throughout climb.	Climbs to the top at a smooth, steady pace and without hesitation.
3	Usually demonstrates essential elements for good technique: a) Maintains 3 points of contact. b) Uses proper foot position. c) Keeps hips close to wall. d) Uses legs to support weight and uses handholds for balance.	Usually executes well-planned movements, with few observable realignments.	Climbs to the top at a smooth, steady pace, with some hesitation.
2	Sometimes demonstrates essential elements for good technique.	Sometimes moves without a plan; wastes motion, with frequent adjustments in holds and alignment; and displays fatigue.	Climbs with several stops, gets only half-way to the top or loses contact with the wall.
1	Seldom demonstrates essential elements for good technique.	Seldom moves with a plan. Body motion is inefficient; shows no evidence of planned movements.	Climbs with several stops and does not reach half-way to the top.
0	Violates safety procedures and/or does not complete the assessment task.		

Scoring: Consistently = 90% or above; Usually = 75% – 89% of the time; Sometimes = 50% – 74%; Seldom = below 50%

■ **Assessment Protocols:**

Directions for Students (Read aloud, verbatim):

- You will be asked to top-rope free-climb a 20-foot vertical wall of an intermediate level of difficulty.

- You should complete the climb using efficient movements and with as little assistance from your belay as possible.

- You will be assessed on your ability to:

  a) Maintain 3 points of contact at all times.

  b) Use proper foot position.

  c) Keep hips close to the wall.

  d) Use legs to support weight and use handholds for balance.

  e) Execute well-planned movements, with few observable realignments.

  f) Climb to the top with a steady pace.

- Touch the 20-foot mark before descending.

- Follow all safety rules.

Directions for Teachers:
Preparation:

- See the chapter titled Administering & Scoring PE Metrics Assessments for instruction and warm-up.

- Film only one student at a time.

- Do not coach the student during the assessment.

- If two climbing walls are available and easily viewable on the video camera, you may assess 2 students at one time.

Safety:

- Check the conditions of the wall, ropes and personal gear before students begin their climbs.

- A trained and attentive belayer should be used for each climber.

- Verbal safety commands between climber and belay should be used at all times.

Equipment/Materials:

- Students should climb only on a well-maintained wall or outdoor course.

- Equipment should be checked frequently for defects and wear and tear.

- Numbered pinnies.

Diagram of Space/Distances:

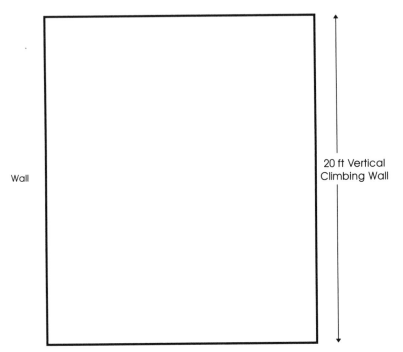

Wall

20 ft Vertical
Climbing Wall

Student

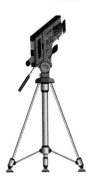

Camera Location/Operation:

Place the camera in an elevated position; preferably, 10 feet off the floor at a 45-degree angle from the student start position on the wall. The top and bottom of the wall should be visible in the camera view as close as possible.

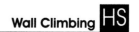

Assessment Score Sheet

PE Teacher _____   Grade _____   Date _____

School _____   Classroom Teacher _____

Pinnie Number	Student Name	Gender	Grade	Technique (0-4)	Body Efficiency (0-4)	Complete Climb (0-4)	Total Score (0-12) 9=Competent

HS Weight Training

Standard 1:

Demonstrates competency in motor skills and movement patterns needed to perform a variety of physical activities.

Performance Indicator:

Demonstrate competency in individual noncompetitive activities.

Assessment Task:

Perform and spot a bench press (free weight) exercise for 5-10 repetitions, demonstrating safe equipment handling and the ability to use correct lifting and spotting techniques.

Criteria for Competence (Level 3):

1. 1 error in essential elements of safety.
2. 1 error in lifting technique.
3. Demonstrates all essential elements of spotting technique.

■ Assessment Rubric:

Level	1. Safety	2. Lifting	3. Spotting
4	No errors in essential elements of safety.	Uses all the essential elements of lifting technique.	No errors in spotting technique; clearly safety-conscious & attentive.
3	1 error in essential elements of safety.	1 error in lifting technique.	Demonstrates all essential elements of spotting technique.
2	2 errors in safety.	2 errors in lifting technique.	Does not appear ready, does not provide assistance when needed/ required or uses 1 essential element of correct technique incorrectly.
1	More than 2 errors in safety.	More than 2 errors in lifting technique.	Does not appear ready, does not provide assistance when needed/ required *and* uses more than 1 essential element of correct technique incorrectly.
0	Violates safety procedures and/or does not complete the assessment task.		

Essential Elements of Weight Training:
Safety

    A. Loads bar evenly.

    B. Secures clips.

    C. Removes and returns weights and/or clips to the rack.

Lifting

    A. Uses an overhand grip.

    B. Hands at least shoulder-width apart.

    C. Feet on the floor or on the bench to create a flat back.

    D. Wrists straight.

    E. Lowers bar to the chest.

    F. Pushes bar up evenly.

    G. Pauses when elbows are straight.

    H. Uses full range of motion (ROM).

    I. Uses at least 4 seconds to move through range of motion (2 seconds up and 2 seconds down).

Spotting

    A. Is in a ready position to assist if needed.

    B. Recognizes when lifter needs assistance and provides it.

    C. If needed:

        1) Uses an alternate grip.

        2) Thumbs are wrapped.

        3) Hands approximately shoulder-width apart.

        4) Feet and back are straight.

    D. Assists to return bar to the rack.

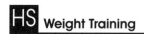

■ **Assessment Protocols:**

Directions for Students (Read aloud, verbatim):

- In this assessment, you will be asked to perform a bench press exercise with a spotter. Use a challenging weight that you can lift for 1 set (5-10 reps).

- You will be assessed on:
  - a) Your safe use of equipment.
  - b) Your ability to use correct lifting techniques.
  - c) Your ability to use correct spotting techniques.

- You will load, lift and break down the equipment by yourself, while your partner serves only as your spotter. Then, your partner will load, lift and break down the equipment, and you will act as his/her spotter.

Directions for Teachers:
Preparation:

- See the chapter titled Administering & Scoring PE Metrics Assessments for instruction and warm-up.

- If multiple benches are used, be sure that all students can be seen clearly from the side angle (~ 45°).

- Students should be paired up with partners similar in size, if possible.

- At no point should students be permitted to continue an exercise that you feel is unsafe.

- Require all students to complete adequate warm-up prior to testing.

Safety:

- Stop the assessment if conditions are unsafe or if improper student techniques deem it unsafe.

Equipment/Materials:

- Free weights that students have used previously or other equipment if free weights are not available.

- Clips should be available and used if assessing on free weights.

- Numbered pinnies.

Diagram of Space/Distances:

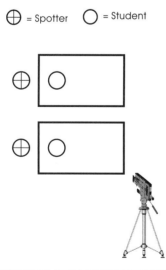

⊕ = Spotter   ◯ = Student

Camera Location/Operation:

The camera should be set up so that both students can be viewed during the performance of set up, one set each, and the break down of the free weight bench press. The testing situation should be set up at the feet to view both students. The student's entire body should be in view and close enough to determine full range of motion, breathing, bar and body placement, grip etc. Depending on the weight room's arrangement it may be possible to video more than one set of students at a time. The camera should stay with one student long enough to video the complete set up, one set of an exercise, and the complete breakdown of equipment.

Assessment Score Sheet

PE Teacher _____   Grade _____   Date _____

School _____   Classroom Teacher _____

Pinnie Number	Student Name	Gender	Grade	Safety (Use/Return Weights & Clips) (0-4)	Lifting (Grip, ROM, Speed) (0-4)	Spotting (Grip, Assistance) (0-4)	Total Score (0-12) 9=Competent

NASPE

Standards 2–6
Performance Descriptors & Sample Questions

This book and the accompanying CD-ROM provide sample assessment questions for National Standards 2-6. The sample questions are divided by performance descriptor so that teachers can select questions based on the content that they've taught their students. Teachers may use entire tests for a standard or may select items across or within particular standards.

PE Metrics: Assessing National Standards 1-6 in Secondary School offers the test items in two different ways:

1. The book offers printed sample question items keyed to specific standards and performance descriptors. Teachers may use these items, especially for formative assessments. *Note:* Correct answers are in **bold** type.

2. The CD-ROM accompanying this book contains the same sample test items and performance descriptors, and teachers are encouraged to copy them into a Word document from which to administer items to students. Answer keys are at the end of each sample test bank.

Note: NASPE's test-writing committees developed no written assessments for kindergarten students because committee members believe that a written test is not appropriate for that grade level.

Teachers from school districts that subscribe to NASPE's PE Metrics Online will have access to different test items, which also are linked to the same standards and performance descriptors. Access to PE Metrics Online, then, doubles the number of test items that teachers have available for using in assessments. In addition, PE Metrics Online users will be able to generate reports for students or parents to explain performance on the test.

Standard 2, Grade 8
Performance Descriptors & Sample Questions

*Editor's note: Correct answers appear in **bold** type.*

Performance Descriptor: Explains critical elements of specialized skills.

Sample Questions

1. To perform a soccer throw-in, which best describes the arm action? Using two hands:
   A. **Take the ball behind the head and follow through toward the receiver's feet.**
   B. Take the ball behind the head and follow through toward the receiver's head.
   C. Bring the ball in to the chest and follow through toward the receiver's feet.
   D. Bring the ball in to the chest and follow through toward the receiver's head.

2. To receive a floor hockey pass, which best describes the action?
   A. Hold the wrists stiff and stop the pass.
   B. Keep the blade open and move it forward on contact.
   C. **Bend the wrists slightly and give with the blade.**
   D. Use a slight backswing and strike the ball or puck as it approaches you.

3. What is the action needed to chip a soccer ball?
   A. **A quick, hard stab under the ball.**
   B. A quick slap at the side of the ball.
   C. A hard kick at the middle of the ball.
   D. A soft slap under the ball.

4. Luis asked you to teach him to shoot a basketball. What critical parts of the release should you tell him?
   A. Push the ball off your palm, keeping your wrist stiff.
   B. Push the ball off your fingers, keeping your wrist stiff.
   C. Push the ball off your palm while snapping your wrist.
   D. **Spin the ball off your fingers while snapping your wrist.**

5. John wants to shoot the soccer ball from farther away. What would you tell him to help him improve?
   A. **Run to the ball, plant the non-kicking foot next to it, and swing your kicking leg way back, with knee bent.**
   B. Stand next to the ball, plant the non-kicking foot next to it, and swing your kicking leg way back, with knee straight.
   C. Run up to the ball faster and kick it, making sure that you follow through high and forward, stepping on the kicking leg.
   D. Leap, plant the non-kicking foot in front of the ball, and swing your kicking leg way back.

6. Paul has asked you to help him with his softball hitting. What would you tell him to help him?
   A. Start with bat slightly back, and make a big chop until bat almost hits the ground in front of you.
   B. Start with bat in front of you. When the ball is released, swing back, then forward in a big scoop.
   C. Start with bat back so that your chin touches your front shoulder. Swing level until your chin is on your back shoulder.
   D. Start with bat back and swing upward until you hit it. Then, drop it.

7. Deepak is trying to throw a Frisbee® in a straight line. Which would help him improve?
   A. Have the disc leave your hand with the side tipped down.
   B. Use a backhand release, with little follow-through.
   C. Have the disc leave your hand with the front tipped up.
   D. Make sure that the disc leaves your hand flat.

Performance Descriptor: Analyzes how positive transfer improves skill performance.

Sample Questions

8. When two skills are similar, and being good at one usually means that you will be good at the other, the skills have:
   A. Negative strategies.
   B. Positive strategies.
   C. Negative transfer.
   D. Positive transfer.

9. What about soccer would help Renee **improve** at Ultimate Frisbee®?
   A. The playing field is the same.
   B. Similar skills are needed.
   C. Offensive and defensive tactics are the same.
   D. Goal-keeping skills are the same.

10. The skills for pickleball will transfer best to which of the following activities:
    A. Frisbee®.
    B. Tennis.
    C. Golf.
    D. Bowling.

11. Which of the following will help Tracy improve a volleyball forearm pass (bump) **most**?
    A. Knowing volleyball rules.
    B. Standing in ready position, as in basketball.
    C. Practicing good teamwork.
    D. Better cardiovascular fitness.

Performance Descriptor: Examines how force and spin can alter the outcomes of skill performance.

Sample Questions

12. To jump for distance, the takeoff angle should be with the body:
    A. **Angled forward.**
    B. Straight up.
    C. Leaning backward.
    D. In a tuck position.

13. How is the rebound on a bounce pass affected by putting topspin on the ball? The bounce will be:
    A. Higher than if no topspin.
    B. The same as if no topspin.
    C. **Faster than if no topspin.**
    D. Slower than if no topspin.

14. When performing a discus throw, a(n)_____ person has an advantage.
    A. Older.
    B. Shorter.
    C. **Taller.**
    D. Younger.

15. Which of the following is **most** likely to produce lift when thrown?
    A. Softball.
    B. Shot put.
    C. **Frisbee®.**
    D. Golf ball.

16. How does Janet produce backspin when hitting a ball? She hits the ball:
    A. At center.
    B. **Below the center.**
    C. Above the center.
    D. Hard anywhere.

Performance Descriptor: Analyzes basic game strategies for invasion (e.g., ultimate, soccer), net (badminton, volleyball) and fielding (softball) games.

Sample Questions

17. Both right-handed players on a doubles tennis team are at the net. The ball comes down the center of the court. Who should take it?
    A. The better player.
    B. The player on the right.
    C. The player with the better forehand.
    D. **The player on the left.**

18. In soccer, the offense has taken a shot and the ball is coming toward the goal. Your goalkeeper and your back could play the ball. Both are equally skilled. Whom do you want to play it?
    A. **The goalkeeper should use hands to play it.**
    B. The back should run up and kick it away.
    C. The back should kick it upfield.
    D. The goalkeeper should kick it upfield while the ball is still on the move.

19. Should offensive players in soccer interchange positions?
    A. No, they are required to stay in the same positions.
    B. Yes, they can use their strongest skills and confuse the defense.
    C. No, they should stay in their positions to keep other players on their team from becoming confused.
    D. Yes, but only after a goal.

20. A basketball player who is guarded closely is attempting to get open for a pass. What should this player do?
    A. Keep moving back and forth until a passing lane opens.
    B. Fake in one direction, cut sharply in the opposite and put one hand out as a target.
    C. Tell your teammate not to throw it in this direction.
    D. Wave hands around and try to distract the defense to create an opening.

21. How does zone defense differ from a player-to-player defense?
    A. Player-to-player defense is more difficult to learn.
    B. Zone defense is more effective against slow players.
    C. Zone defense requires a player to guard an area.
    D. Player-to-player defense requires staying in the same position on the court or field.

22. In which situation should the batter bunt?
    A. No outs with a runner on first.
    B. Two outs with runners on first and third.
    C. Two outs with runners on second and third.
    D. One out with the bases loaded.

Performance Descriptor: Analyzes the role of physical abilities in performance.

Sample Questions

23. A person's physical ability can be defined as:
    A. The result of practice only.
    B. What you are born with and what you learn and practice.
    C. What you are born with only.
    D. How hard you try only.

24. If a person is strong and has a low center of gravity, which sport is he/she likely to master?
    A. Tennis.
    B. Wrestling.
    C. High-jumping.
    D. Swimming.

25. Which physical characteristic can help you become a good basketball player?
    A. Flexibility.
    B. Strength.
    C. Height.
    D. Balance.

26. Size, skill, strength, height and motivation contribute to playing different positions in basketball. Which are most important for a center?
    A. **Height and strength, for working within the key.**
    B. Motivation and skill, for knowing how to score.
    C. Size and height, to move down the court quickly.
    D. Skill and strength, for dribbling up the court.

27. Your little sister, who is in 7th grade, wants to play basketball. She is short, like both of your parents, and practices every day. What will you tell her to help her?
    A. She won't get better even with practice, so she shouldn't play any sport.
    B. She probably will not grow tall, so she should switch to a sport in which height doesn't matter.
    C. **She probably won't grow very tall, so she should practice skills to play a guard position.**
    D. She can keep practicing, but if she isn't good by now, she probably will never be a good basketball player.

28. In basketball, the best players are taller, faster and stronger, and have better skills. Of the following attributes, which can most improve with practice?
    A. Speed.
    B. Height.
    C. Strength.
    D. **Skills.**

Standards 3 & 4, Grade 8
Performance Descriptors & Sample Questions

*Editor's note: Correct answers appear in **bold** type.*

Performance Descriptor: Participates in a variety of physical activities as part of a healthful lifestyle.

Sample Questions

1. Which of the following **best** describes a physically active lifestyle?
   A. Runs a mile at least 2 days a week, takes piano lessons weekly, and walks the dog for 10 minutes every day.
   B. Plays golf, swims regularly and enjoys riding a bike.
   C. Walks a half-mile to and from school 5 days a week and helps with weekly chores at home.
   D. Participates daily in a personal fitness plan and plays in seasonal community sports leagues.

2. Mary performs stretching exercises and runs most days of the week to be able to increase her:
   A. Arm and shoulder strength.
   B. Muscle endurance and abdominal strength.
   C. Flexibility and aerobic endurance.
   D. Flexibility and body weight.

3. Juan's grandfather and father both have a history of heart disease. Juan has decided to try to prevent heart disease. Which of the following describes a lifestyle that would be most healthful?
   A. Completes a personal physical fitness plan most days of the week.
   B. Plays basketball in a community league 2 days a week.
   C. Walks to and from school for a total of 20 minutes each day.
   D. Enjoys roller-skating, biking and hiking on weekends.

4. Which of the following tools is **most** useful for determining the intensity of your workout?
   A. Stop watch.
   B. Digital pedometer.
   C. Calorimeter.
   D. Heart rate monitor.

Performance Descriptor: Demonstrates use of self-management skills related to maintaining a physically active lifestyle.

Sample Questions

5. Which of the following plans is **best** for maintaining a physically active lifestyle?
   A. Try to walk whenever possible, instead of riding in the car.
   B. Write a realistic personal physical activity schedule and follow it.
   C. Participate in some physical activity every weekend.
   D. Record all of your activities every day.

6. Mary enjoys being physically active and participating with her friends but doesn't like competitive activities. Which of the following group of activities is she most likely to include in her plan for physical activity?
   A. **Hiking & jogging.**
   B. Dancing & basketball.
   C. Swimming & dancing.
   D. Tennis & archery.

Performance Descriptor: Participates in a variety of health-enhancing fitness activities to improve health-related physical fitness.

Sample Questions

7. Which group of activities is **most** likely to improve your overall health-related physical fitness?
   A. Swimming, biking & running.
   B. Using weight machines & free weights.
   C. **Walking/jogging, stretching & weight training.**
   D. Stretching, volleyball & softball.

8. Improving muscle strength requires completing a workout that includes:
   A. Running a mile at least 2 times a week.
   B. Stretching major muscles at least 1 time a week.
   C. Practicing 100-yard sprints every day of the week.
   D. **Lifting weights at least 3 times a week.**

9. Which of the following is **most** likely to help maintain one's health-related physical fitness?
   A. Participating in activities that require balance, coordination and agility at least 3 days a week.
   B. **Completing a workout that includes cardiovascular, weight-lifting and stretching exercises at least 5 days a week.**
   C. Participating in school intramural or pick-up sports with friends at least 3 days a week.
   D. Participating in activities that increase heart rate and breathing at least 2 days a week.

Performance Descriptor: Evaluates current level of physical activity.

Sample Question

10. You have kept a log of your physical activity for one week and have discovered that, on school days, you get little or no moderate-to-vigorous physical activity. Which of the following will **best** help to increase your level of physical activity?
    A. Perform additional chores at home at least 2 days a week.
    B. Work out more vigorously on weekends.
    C. **Plan and participate in specific moderate-to-vigorous physical activity each day.**
    D. Do everything on your schedule faster.

Performance Descriptor: Achieves healthy levels of health-related, criterion-referenced standards for fitness.

Sample Questions

11. A test of health-related fitness that **best** provides information about your level of physical fitness includes the following:
    A. Balance, coordination & body composition.
    B. Reaction time, agility & balance.
    C. Aerobic endurance, reaction time & speed.
    D. Aerobic endurance, flexibility & muscle endurance.

12. John scored very low on a test of his aerobic fitness. Which of the following would **best** help him improve his score on this test?
    A. Walking fast or jogging at least a mile most days of the week.
    B. Performing exercises to strengthen arm and shoulder muscles every other day.
    C. Including stretching and curl-up exercises in his daily workout.
    D. Participating in activities that require coordination, agility and reaction time

Performance Descriptor: Applies principles of training to improve and/or maintain the specific components of health-related fitness.

Sample Questions

13. A fitness plan to improve aerobic fitness should include:
    A. Activities that make the arm and shoulder muscles tired and that are performed 3 days a week.
    B. Activities that are competitive and that are performed 2 days a week.
    C. Activities that help decrease the resting heart rate at least 3 days a week.
    D. Activities that increase and maintain the heart rate in the target heart rate zone for 30 minutes each day.

14. Mary's typical weekly physical activity plan includes a 30-minute run at least 5 days of the week. Which component of fitness is **most** likely to improve with this plan?
    A. Agility.
    B. Reaction time.
    C. Aerobic endurance.
    D. Coordination.

15. Flexibility and aerobic endurance improvements require performing specific exercises:
    A. Most days of the week.
    B. Once a week.
    C. Two days per week.
    D. Three days per week.

16. Performing weight-training exercises using correct technique, a slow lift and let-down and always moving through the full range of motion are important guidelines for improving:
    A. Aerobic endurance.
    B. Muscle endurance.
    C. Reaction time & balance.
    D. Coordination & agility.

17. A muscle-endurance workout requires _____ than a muscle-strength workout.
    A. Lifting more weight for fewer numbers of repetitions.
    B. Performing the workout fewer times a week.
    C. Lifting less weight for more repetitions.
    D. Performing more sets in each workout.

18. The **most** important element in planning your workout is:
    A. What you do after your workout.
    B. Setting realistic goals based on your fitness test scores.
    C. How long your workout should last.
    D. How often you can work out.

Performance Descriptor: Assesses physiological indicators of exercise during and after physical activity.

Sample Questions

19. You can determine the intensity of a physical activity by:
    A. Measuring time, distance or heart rate achieved during an activity period.
    B. Keeping a log of daily physical activities.
    C. Following a physical activity plan.
    D. Counting the number of participants in the activity.

20. The part of a physical activity that prepares the body for moderate-to-vigorous activity is the:
    A. Workout.
    B. Cool-down.
    C. Warm-up.
    D. Rest period.

21. Which of the following activities is **best** to use as both a warm-up and cool-down?
    A. Juggling.
    B. Rope-jumping.
    C. Weight-lifting exercises.
    D. Walking.

22. The warm-up and cool-down are performed before and after a vigorous workout to:
    A. Increase the amount of time that you can work out.
    B. Regulate blood flow and body temperature.
    C. Determine how much weight you can lift.
    D. Increase the distance that you can run.

23. When performing a muscle-strength or muscle-endurance workout, you should:
    A. Rest for 30 to 60 seconds between each set.
    B. Perform only one set each workout day.
    C. Change the exercise and muscles used after each set.
    D. Rest for 10 minutes before starting a new exercise.

Performance Descriptor: Describes the relationship of cardiorespiratory fitness, muscle strength and endurance, and flexibility to body composition.

Sample Questions

24. The **most** effective physical activities for losing fat are:
    A. Bowling & hiking.
    B. Walking & cleaning.
    C. Stretching & skating.
    D. Running & jogging.

25. Which of the following is considered the **most** healthy lifestyle and is personally controllable?
    A. Regular moderate-to-vigorous physical activity.
    B. Watching television for several hours each day.
    C. Using tobacco, illegal drugs & alcohol.
    D. Overeating and limiting physical activity.

26. The relationship of fat to lean tissue is a factor that is used to determine:
    A. Flexibility.
    B. Body composition.
    C. Muscle strength.
    D. Aerobic capacity.

Performance Descriptor: Applies principles of conditioning that enhance performance.

Sample Questions

27. Bob is a distance runner on the track team and wants to improve his time in the 800-meter run. His conditioning program should include:
    A. Arm- and shoulder-strength exercises.
    B. Running increasingly longer distances.
    C. Long intervals of rest.
    D. Flexibility exercises.

28. You can improve your overall performance in a specific activity by:
    A. Practicing with less-skilled opponents.
    B. Participating in variety of physical activities.
    C. Improving your fitness level in those factors that the activity requires.
    D. Practicing isolated parts of skills and skill combinations.

29. A training program for game performance includes a combination of high-quality skill practice and a workout plan to maintain personal levels of health-related fitness, including:
    A. Aerobic & muscle endurance.
    B. Height & weight.
    C. Coordination & reaction time.
    D. Flexibility & balance.

Standards 5 & 6, Grade 8
Performance Descriptors & Sample Questions

*Editor's note: Correct answers appear in **bold** type.*

Performance Descriptor: Applies procedures for keeping others and self safe during physical activity.

Sample Questions

1. You're hiking with your friends and one of them can't keep up with the rest. You should:
   A. Ask that friend to wait at a spot until you return.
   B. Ask for a volunteer to stay back with the slower friend on the hike.
   C. **Adjust the pace of your hike to meet the needs of your slow friend.**
   D. Stop hiking and turn back so that all of you can be together.

2. Your class is lifting weights and you notice that Bob never lets his spotter do what he is supposed to do. What should you do?
   A. Ignore it, so long as you think Bob can handle the situation.
   B. **Tell Bob that he needs to let the spotter do his job to be safe.**
   C. Tell the teacher that Bob isn't using his spotter.
   D. Tell the spotter to spot regardless of what Bob wants.

Performance Descriptor: Describes problem-solving techniques to resolve conflicts.

Sample Questions

3. If you're practicing with a partner who is not very good at the volleyball set and is not even trying to be good, what should you do?
   A. Send the ball to your partner the way he/she sent it to you.
   B. **Ask your partner to give you a set that is playable.**
   C. Tell the teacher.
   D. Stop practicing with the partner until he/she gets the idea about what he/she is supposed to do.

4. You and your partner are assessing each other at the end of a tennis unit. Your partner asks you to record a score that she did not earn. What should you do?
   A. Do what your partner says so that you don't create conflict, and let the teacher handle it.
   B. **Ignore your partner's request and record the correct score.**
   C. Tell the teacher.
   D. Do what your partner says but take points off the next part of the test.

5. Resolving a conflict over an out-of-bounds ball in a sport is best accomplished by:
   A. Ignoring the disagreement.
   B. Asking an adult to solve the problem.
   C. **Declaring a "do-over."**
   D. Giving the other team the advantage on the next out-of-bounds ball.

6. When you're playing a game with a student referee and you think he/she doesn't know a rule, what should you do?
   A. Nothing; accept the calls as they are made.
   B. Share the correct rule with the referee.
   C. Accept the referee's call and ask him/her about it later.
   D. Ask for a "do-over."

7. If one person on your team insists at yelling to give him the ball, what should you do?
   A. Give it to him if he's a good player.
   B. Don't pass him the ball, so that he learns to be quiet.
   C. Yell for him to pass the ball to you when he has it.
   D. Ask him not to yell and he will get his share of the plays.

8. If a student calls you a bad name while playing a game, what should you do?
   A. Call the student a bad name, and keep playing.
   B. Try to ignore the student and keep playing but get back at him/her later.
   C. Stop playing and tell the teacher.
   D. Say "I don't like being called a bad name; I wouldn't say that to you" and keep playing.

9. During class, you and your friends are having a good time in the group to which you were assigned but you're not really paying attention to the teacher. You realize that your behavior is not correct. What should you do?
   A. Stop your behavior immediately and find another group.
   B. Continue until the teacher tells you to stop.
   C. Remind your friends that all of you need to stop what you're doing.
   D. Pay attention to the teacher and don't worry about what the group is doing.

Performance Descriptor: Demonstrates concern for the rights and feelings of others in resolving conflicts.

Sample Questions

10. Which of the following is the **best** example of good sportsmanship?
    A. Letting the other team win some points so that it doesn't fall so far behind.
    B. Not celebrating after the game when you win.
    C. Giving feedback to the other team on what it might do to play better.
    D. Congratulating your opponents on a good win when you lose.

11. You're playing a pickup game of softball with your friends. You hit the ball and run to first base. Your team calls you "safe," even though you know you were not. What should you do?
    A. Let the two teams work it out and don't say anything.
    B. Admit to your team that you were out.
    C. Tell both teams that the matter needs to be resolved with a "do-over."
    D. Agree with your team.

12. You can best support classmates who are not good at an activity by:
    A. Telling them that they really are not as bad as they think they are.
    B. Taking their turns so that they don't have to do it and look bad.
    C. Not laughing when they make a mistake.
    D. Giving them positive feedback when they do well.

Performance Descriptor: Exhibits supportive verbal and nonverbal behavior toward peers of different gender, race, ethnicity and ability.

Sample Questions

13. When someone deliberately pushes you in a game, you should:
    A. Continue to play and not worry about it.
    B. Wait until the official or someone else sees it before doing anything.
    C. Push him/her back, but not as hard.
    D. Ask the person to stop in a firm but not-threatening voice.

14. If you're asked to complete a group assignment but none of your friends are in your group, what should you do?
    A. Do your fair share of the work and support the efforts of the group members.
    B. Stay with the group but don't participate enthusiastically, so that the teacher knows you're not happy.
    C. Ask the teacher to put you in another group.
    D. Switch places with a person in the group that you want to be with.

15. When you've clearly done something that you know you're not supposed to do and your teacher brings it to your attention, you should:
    A. Explain to the teacher why you did it.
    B. Ask the teacher to enforce the rule on others in the group who are doing the same thing.
    C. Discuss with the teacher why you think it's a bad rule.
    D. Acknowledge that you did it and say that it won't happen again.

16. If your teacher assigns you to a partner who is much better than you in an activity, what should you do?
    A. Tell your partner that he/she might want to ask the teacher for a new partner.
    B. Ask the partner for some help in improving.
    C. Try not to let the partner know that you're not very good.
    D. Explain to your partner why you don't like the activity.

17. One of the biggest reasons that a classmate might not show much effort when asked to participate with you in a physical activity is that he/she:
    A. Just doesn't like to be physically active.
    B. Would rather have a different partner.
    C. Probably isn't good at the activity and doesn't want to look bad.
    D. Thinks he/she is already good at the activity.

18. You are **not** working productively with your partner when you:
    A. Take your partner's turn to serve when you know that he/she is having trouble serving.
    B. Give your partner more chances than you have to practice.
    C. Give your partner feedback on his/her performance.
    D. Throw him/her the ball so that he/she can succeed.

Performance Descriptor: Values participating in physical activity because of the health benefits, personal enjoyment and/or social interaction.

Sample Question

19. What would be the easiest lifestyle change that would improve your level of physical activity?
    A. Taking the stairs instead of the elevator.
    B. Signing up for karate lessons after school.
    C. Playing on a sport team after school.
    D. Participating in a running program before school.

Performance Descriptor: Recognizes competition as a source of challenge.

Sample Questions

20. If a person is good at an activity, he/she probably:
    A. Was born good at it.
    B. Has parents who are good at it.
    C. Is good at most activities.
    D. Has practiced the activity a lot.

21. If you want a highly competitive aerobic challenge, you should choose to:
    A. Participate during archery class.
    B. Play 18 holes of golf for both days of a weekend.
    C. Train for monthly YMCA fun runs.
    D. Compete in a weekly bowling league.

Performance Descriptor: Identifies personal preferences (e.g., enjoyment, fun, social interaction) as criteria for selecting physical activities.

Sample Questions

22. People are most likely to participate in activities that:
    A. Are competitive.
    B. Allow boys and girls to play together.
    C. Don't take a lot of time.
    D. They are good at.

23. If you're deciding what physical activities to try, which of the following ways should you choose new activities?
    A. Choose activities that you can do at home.
    B. Select activities that require a long-term commitment so that you can stay active.
    C. Select activities that your friends participate in.
    D. Select activities that are exciting, fun or challenging for you.

24. If Wendy likes risk-taking challenges and wants to develop upper-body strength, which activity should she select?
    A. Rock climbing.
    B. Playing golf.
    C. Water aerobics.
    D. Tennis.

Standard 2, High School
Performance Descriptors & Sample Questions

*Editor's note: Correct answers appear in **bold** type.*

Performance Descriptor: Compares/contrasts critical elements of specialized skills originating from a common movement pattern.

Sample Questions:

1. The overhand-throw pattern is very similar to which of the following?
   A. Discus throw.
   B. Pickleball serve.
   C. Tennis serve.
   D. Soccer throw-in.

2. Which movement pattern is most similar to the bowling release?
   A. Badminton serve.
   B. Softball underhand pitch.
   C. Volleyball forearm pass.
   D. Floor or ice hockey pass.

3. The tennis forehand and badminton forehand are similar in many ways. In what way are they different?
   A. In tennis, you keep the wrist firm; but in badminton, you snap the wrist on release.
   B. In tennis, you snap the wrist on release; but in badminton, you keep your wrist firm.
   C. In tennis, you contact the ball at the baseline; but in badminton, you hit closer to the net.
   D. In tennis, you're trying to win the point; but in badminton, you try to keep a volley going.

4. The basketball guarding position and the volleyball serve-receive position are similar in many ways, but in what way are they different?
   A. In basketball, your weight is low; but in volleyball you stand up.
   B. In basketball, one arm usually is up; but in volleyball, both are low.
   C. In basketball, you're on your toes; but in volleyball, you're on your heels.
   D. They're the same, except that you try to hit a volleyball and catch a basketball.

5. From the following list of skills, what are the similarities? Football pass, softball throw from the outfield, tennis serve, badminton smash.
   A. There are no similarities; they are discrete skills.
   B. All are offensive skills.
   C. All are skills that require height for success.
   D. All use an overhand-throw pattern.

6. A badminton serve is different from a softball hit because it is a:
   A. Striking pattern, but it is overhead.
   B. Striking pattern but it is sidearm.
   C. Striking pattern, but it is underhand.
   D. Striking pattern, but the person is moving.

Performance Descriptor: Designs advanced game strategies for invasion, net, fielding and target activities.

Sample Questions:

7. When playing softball, it's best to hit a sacrifice fly when:
   A. A runner is on 3rd base, with less than two outs.
   B. No runners are on base, with less than two outs.
   C. The bases are loaded, with two outs.
   D. A runner is on 1st base, with one out.

8. The best time to use a zone defense in soccer is when:
   A. The opponents are very slow and have weak soccer skills.
   B. The opponents are too fast to keep up with and can control the ball well.
   C. You're tired or the goalkeeper is hurt.
   D. You have no substitutes to fill in for you.

9. Your volleyball team has the following people in the back row: the tallest hitter, the setter & the defensive specialist. Which one should take the second hit?
   A. The defensive specialist.
   B. The hitter.
   C. The setter.
   D. Whomever the ball is hit to.

10. Your opponent in tennis has an excellent net game. What strategy should you use?
    A. Hit all returns deep and to the corners.
    B. Vary your shots, with lobs and short shots.
    C. Hit the ball hard and to the middle of the court.
    D. Any defensive strategy will work.

11. On your soccer team, you have a very weak goalkeeper and one very skilled forward. It's near the end of the game and you have a 1-goal lead. The opponents have just made a pass deep into the corner near your goal. What do you do?
    A. Line up a "wall" near the goal line.
    B. Kick it to your goalkeeper to kick back.
    C. Leave it until your forward comes to get it.
    D. Try to clear it well down the field.

12. In softball, you have a runner on 1st and 2nd bases with 2 outs and the score tied. Where should you try to hit the ball to have the greatest opportunity to advance the runner on 2nd base?
    A. Grounder into right field.
    B. Grounder to left field.
    C. Grounder to 3rd base.
    D. Deep fly ball to center field.

Performance Descriptor: Analyzes skill performance using biomechanical concepts.

Sample Questions:

13. Rosa is trying to kick a ball as far as possible, but with no success. She should make sure that she has a full range of motion by using:
    A. A short backswing and a full follow-through.
    B. A full backswing and a full follow-through.
    C. No backswing and a full follow-through.
    D. A full backswing and a short follow-through.

14. It's important when throwing a ball to step forward on the opposite foot, because that provides:
    A. Stability and increased lever length.
    B. Momentum, and it shortens the range of motion.
    C. Momentum and maximum preparation to rotate.
    D. Stability and decreased lever length.

15. A discus thrower is not getting much distance on his/her throws. What can you suggest to help increase the distance?
    A. Extend the arm fully at the end of the rotation and release as the arm moves up to shoulder height.
    B. Keep the arm wrapped around the body at the end of the rotation and release as high as possible.
    C. Work on upper-body strength training to build arm bulk.
    D. Shorten the rotation and release using more arm muscles.

16. A golf ball stops rolling due to friction because:
    A. An object in motion remains in motion until acted upon by an outside force.
    B. For every action, there is an equal and opposite reaction.
    C. Force equals mass times acceleration.
    D. Drag increases with the square of the velocity.

Performance Descriptor: Designs and justifies a practice plan using motor learning concepts.

Sample Questions:

17. Once Satoshi has learned the basic skills in soccer, what kind of practice will help him improve each skill and his overall game performance? Practicing each skill:
    A. On different days to focus only on that one skill.
    B. In a full game of soccer.
    C. Separately but in game-like activities.
    D. Separately, but in isolation activities.

18. Bob wants to learn to play volleyball, and is willing to practice. What is the best practice plan for learning to play the game?
    A. Practice the skills in game-like conditions first and then break the skills down to simple practice conditions.
    B. Practice all skills for some time on each day.
    C. Practice one skill on one day until you're good at it and another skill on another day.
    D. Practice the skills in a game.

19. Which of the following is an open skill that one should practice in game-like conditions?
   A. Basketball free throw.
   B. Batting in softball or baseball.
   C. Soccer dribble.
   D. Tennis serve.

20. Maya is fairly skilled at her sport and wants to try out for her school team. How should she practice on most days to prepare for try-outs?
   A. Work on basic skills, then combine the skills, then play games.
   B. Work on playing in games as much as she can.
   C. Work on each skill separately and then play games.
   D. Work only on those skills she is weak in to use her time more wisely.

Performance Descriptor: Analyzes physical development across the lifespan that influences physical activity choices.

Sample Questions:

21. Which of the following is the most accurate statement about physical activity levels?
   A. If children are not physically active, they won't be physically active when they are adults.
   B. Physical activity patterns stay the same as people age.
   C. Children and older adults are not that physically active.
   D. Physical activity patterns change as people age.

22. A person's size and strength should be considered when choosing:
   A. Sport equipment.
   B. Friends to play with.
   C. The type of sports clothes to buy.
   D. What to drink during activity.

23. Which of the following is true about high school students? They have _____ than elementary students.
   A. Longer limbs, more efficient lungs and similar muscle mass.
   B. Longer limbs, similar lung size and more muscle mass.
   C. Longer limbs, larger lungs and more muscle mass.
   D. Similar-length limbs, equally efficient lungs and more muscle fibers.

24. As people mature and begin to balance job, family and recreation pursuits, their choice of physical activity typically includes more:
   A. Individual and dual activities.
   B. Highly competitive activities.
   C. Large-group activities.
   D. Longer games and sports.

25. Tommy's grandmother played basketball while growing up and still rides a bike and walks regularly. All of the following are benefits that Tommy's grandmother could realize from physical activity, except:
   A. She sleeps better.
   B. She strengthened her bones to help resist osteoporosis.
   C. She has sore muscles.
   D. She has stronger heart and lungs.

26. Mohammad is ahead of his peers in terms of motor skill development, which may be because of more:
    A. Maturity and practice.
    B. Instruction and speed.
    C. Practice, instruction and body size.
    D. Instruction, practice and maturity.

27. As you continue to mature, which of the following is most likely to happen?
    A. I will get faster and stronger as I grow older, and that affects my skills.
    B. My skills will stay the same if I continue to practice.
    C. My skills in most activities will increase if I practice.
    D. My skills will be better immediately.

Standards 3 & 4, High School
Performance Descriptors & Sample Questions

*Editor's note: Correct answers appear in **bold** type.*

Performance Descriptor: Implements a personal physical activity plan that is part of a healthful lifestyle.

Sample Questions

1. A pedometer is usually used to record how physically active you are by:
   A. Recording your peddling action while you ride your bike.
   B. Measuring your average heart rate while you walk.
   C. Counting the number of steps you take during physical activity.
   D. Recording the number of physical activities in which you participate weekly.

2. Amy goes to school, does chores and homework and works as a waitress on weekends. Which would provide the most beneficial physical activity to be worked into her tight schedule?
   A. Walking to school and working at least two days a week.
   B. Performing a long physical activity workout once a week.
   C. Walking as quickly as possible while waitressing.
   D. Performing a personal fitness workout at least 5 days a week.

3. Which one of the following activities is both non-competitive and a proven moderate-to-vigorous physical activity?
   A. Gardening.
   B. Soccer.
   C. Golf.
   D. Archery.

4. You should choose activities for your personal physical activity plan that:
   A. You can fit into your schedule.
   B. You can perform with enjoyment.
   C. Your friends enjoy doing.
   D. Are provided by your local recreation program.

Performance Descriptor: Employs self-management skills to maintain a physically active lifestyle.

Sample Questions

5. Which of the following are benefits of being physically fit?
   A. Decreased heart rate and appetite.
   B. Improved self-esteem and reduced stress.
   C. Increased resting heart rate and lowered stress.
   D. More energy and less need for sleep.

6. A physically active person accumulates up to 60 minutes a day of moderate-to-vigorous physical activity. Which of the following best describes a "physically active lifestyle?"
   A. **Walks to school, mows grass and rakes leaves, cleans house, completes a personal fitness workout 5 to 6 days a week, plays on the school tennis team.**
   B. Rides the bus to school, participates in PE class 2 days a week, works at the local grocery store stocking shelves on weekends.
   C. Completes homework each day, completes chores at home, practices daily with the marching band at school, walks to school.
   D. Participates in a bowling league 1 to 2 days a week, volunteers at the community library restocking books 2 to 3 days a week, runs a mile 3 days a week.

7. Which of the following plans demonstrates the most physically active lifestyle?
   A. Work out at the local fitness center at least 3 days a week.
   B. **Swim or play soccer or tennis for 60 minutes at least 5 days a week.**
   C. Run a mile at least 2 days a week.
   D. Perform a weight-lifting program at least 3 days a week.

8. Which group of activities would most likely help to improve all components of health-related physical fitness if added to your personal physical activity plan?
   A. Biking, volleyball, swimming.
   B. Soccer, basketball, softball.
   C. Gymnastics, running, bowling.
   D. **Yoga, weight lifting, running.**

9. Which group of activities is considered sedentary?
   A. **Reading, schoolwork, writing a paper.**
   B. Rowing, sit-ups, watching a basketball game.
   C. Biking, golf, archery.
   D. Treading water, reading, canoeing.

Performance Descriptor: Achieves levels of health-related criterion-referenced standards for fitness.

Sample Questions

10. The percentages of fat, muscle, bone and water in the body are fitness components called:
    A. Weight management.
    B. Nutritional balance.
    C. **Body composition.**
    D. Physical structure.

11. Running for distance or time can be used to measure:
    A. Flexibility.
    B. **Aerobic endurance.**
    C. Distance capacity.
    D. Muscle strength.

12. Which activity is the **best** measure of arm strength?
    A. **Bent-arm hang.**
    B. Shoulder stretch.
    C. Jumping jacks.
    D. Arm lift.

13. What 2 tests are intended to measure aerobic fitness?
    A. Stress test, sit-ups.
    B. Shoulder stretch, mile run.
    C. Mile run, PACER.
    D. Shuttle run, step test.

Performance Descriptor: Demonstrates the skill, knowledge and desire to monitor and adjust activity levels to meet personal fitness needs.

Sample Questions

14. You can increase the intensity of your workout by:
    A. Increasing distance & speed.
    B. Decreasing speed & distance.
    C. Increasing time & decreasing distance.
    D. Increasing time & decreasing repetitions.

15. In the FITT guidelines, "frequency" refers to:
    A. How long you exercise.
    B. How much time you allow between repetitions.
    C. How often you exercise.
    D. The number of weeks in a workout plan.

16. When you reach your initial goal for improved physical fitness, you should apply the principle of "progression" to safely adjust your work-out plan to continue fitness improvement by:
    A. Increasing the intensity of your workout.
    B. Increasing the number of "no-workout" days per week.
    C. Keeping your workout the same.
    D. Work out at a lower level of intensity.

17. The type of activities to improve aerobic endurance must be able to _____ throughout the activity.
    A. Keep the heart rate at the target heart rate level.
    B. Keep the heart rate at a resting level.
    C. Change the heart rate.
    D. Allow the heart rate to recover.

18. My goal is to lose weight safely and decrease my percentage of body fat in the next four weeks by _____.
    A. Walking daily, reducing water consumption, eating more whole grain bread and eliminating fatty foods.
    B. Walking 30 minutes daily, eating more fruit and vegetables, and consuming more water and fewer calories.
    C. Jogging every other day, avoiding meat and bread, eating more fruit, and drinking 8 glasses of water each day.
    D. Walking 3 times per week, cutting my calorie intake by 25 percent, eating more protein, and increasing my water intake daily.

19. My goal is to complete the mile run without stopping to rest by doing the following for four weeks:

    A. **Alternately run and walk at least 5 days a week, increasing the distance I run gradually.**
    B. Walk briskly for 1¼ miles at least 5 days a week.
    C. Alternately run and walk at least every other day.
    D. Walk 1 mile briskly 3 days the first week and add ½ mile each week after that.

20. You can improve your current level of shoulder flexibility by:

    A. Stretching during warm-up twice per week.
    B. Participating in activities that require a full range of motion twice per week.
    C. **Completing a specific shoulder-flexibility training workout every day.**
    D. Starting all workouts with flexibility training 3 times a week.

21. Sean was able to perform 20 curl-ups on a test for muscle endurance. His goal, within the next six weeks, is to perform 30 curl-ups without resting. Which of the following plans will **best** help to safely improve his score?

    A. **Every other day, complete 3 sets of up to 15 curl-ups each set, with a 1-minute rest between sets.**
    B. Three times a week, perform 3 sets of up to 10 curl-ups each set, with a no rest between sets.
    C. Once a week, perform 3 sets of up to 15 curl-ups each set, with a 1-minute rest between sets.
    D. Once a week, complete the curl-up test, adding 2 curl-ups on each trial for 6 weeks.

22. When planning your exercise program, you should start by:

    A. Using a plan of physical fitness activities based on nationally set goals.
    B. Keeping a log of your participation in all physical activities.
    C. **Reviewing your personal fitness test scores and setting personal fitness goals.**
    D. Deciding how much time you have to exercise.

23. When the length of a run is changed from 1 mile to 1¼ miles, what principle is being applied?

    A. Intensity.
    B. Specificity.
    C. Frequency.
    D. **Progression.**

24. Factors of age and maximum heart rate are two of several items used to determine your:

    A. **Target heart rate zone.**
    B. Aerobic capacity.
    C. Resting heart rate.
    D. Oxygen capacity.

25. When adjusting your workout to increase flexibility, stretch each muscle group beyond the distance required by your normal activities and until:

    A. You cannot stand the pain.
    B. **The muscle becomes tight without painful discomfort.**
    C. You reach the recommended distance for your age group.
    D. Your reach your long-term goal distance.

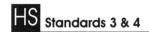

26. A personal fitness workout plan for improving total health-related fitness should include goals based on:
    A. Personal evaluation, with specific activities to address body composition.
    B. Published charts of expectations for a person of your height and weight, with specific activities to address all fitness components.
    C. **Personal test results, specific activities to address each component, and realistic expectations.**
    D. Personal test results and desired achievement of specific sports skills.

Scenario: Goal-Setting. Use to answer questions 27 & 28.

Jamal wants to set up a fitness plan that will improve his fitness levels. He is 15 years old and is in high school. He appears to be healthy but is overweight. Below are his pre-test scores and goals for his fitness plan. Read the goals and answer the questions below.

Jamal's Goals for September through January 31.

Fitness Component	Pre-Test	Goal
Muscle endurance	Push-ups = 1	3
	Curl-ups = 12	20+
Body composition	32% body fat	32% body fat or less
Aerobic endurance	22-minute mile	18-minute mile

27. Jamal has set a goal for improving his push-up score. Which of the following work-out plans is most likely to help him reach his goal?
    A. **Complete 3 sets of up to 10 modified push-ups each, with hands on a table and feet on the floor, every other day for 3 weeks.**
    B. Complete 3 sets of up to 10 modified push-ups each, with hands on a table and feet on the floor, at least 2 days a week for 3 weeks.
    C. Complete 3 sets of up to 10 modified push-ups each, with hands on a table and feet on the floor, at least once a week for 3 weeks.
    D. Complete as many push-ups as you can 3 days a week for 3 weeks.

28. Jamal has set a goal of improving his curl-up score by completing 3 sets of up to 10 curl-ups each, every other day for 3 weeks. If he reaches his goal of 20 curl-ups without rest, Jamal should adjust the goal and continue the workout for 3 more weeks, but:
    A. **Increase the number of repetitions to up to 15 in each set.**
    B. Keep the number of repetitions in each set the same.
    C. Decrease the number of repetitions and increase the number of sets in each workout.
    D. Complete as many curl-ups as possible in each workout.

29. When designing a conditioning program to improve health-related fitness, you should first look at your current fitness test scores to determine realistic goals around which to create a workout plan. Which set of guidelines must you consider for each of the activities/exercises in the daily plan?

   A. Frequency, intensity, time and specific type of exercise needed to address each health-related fitness component.

   B. Personal needs for sleeping, studying, working and eating.

   C. Your physical activity level and interests.

   D. Nutrition needs and eating habits.

Standards 5 & 6, High School
Performance Descriptors & Sample Questions

*Editor's note: Correct answers appear in **bold** type.*

Performance Descriptor: Describes appropriate leadership and followership behaviors.

Sample Questions

1. If Janice is the leader of a group that has chosen a possible solution to a problem, how should she act if she disagrees with the group's decision?
   A. **Accept the decision and try the idea.**
   B. Keep trying to persuade the group to select her idea.
   C. Ask the person who recommended the chosen plan to take over being leader.
   D. Remind group members that she is the leader and that they should do what she thinks is best.

2. If your team is losing most of your games, the best action for the team leader would be to:
   A. Tell the team that winning isn't everything.
   B. **Work with the team to determine where the problems are.**
   C. Discipline team members when they don't practice hard.
   D. Create a strategy to hide less-skilled players.

3. Good leaders:
   A. Keep all members in line.
   B. Solve problems before anyone else in the group knows a problem exists.
   C. **Make everyone feel part of a group.**
   D. Make sure that everyone knows to follow directions.

4. Casey was chosen as captain of his team and is supposed to lead the practice before a game. He knows what to do but is afraid that the team will not follow him. He should:
   A. Skip the practice and move on to something else until he feels as though the group is with him.
   B. Ask someone else to lead the practice.
   C. Ask group members whether they want to undertake the practice he planned.
   D. **Tell group members what they will be doing, and begin the practice.**

5. Jason loves to dance and is thrilled when the rhythm unit begins. Most of his classmates are afraid of what they might look like while dancing. He should:
   A. Help his classmates by correcting their mistakes.
   B. Suggest that his classmates ask the teacher not to do a dance unit.
   C. Suggest to the teacher that non-dancers just watch if they want to.
   D. **Promote that the idea is to have fun and you don't have to be the perfect dancer.**

Performance Descriptor: Applies problem-solving techniques.

Sample Question

6. If Matt has the solution to a problem that his group is trying to answer, he should:
    A. Tell the group the answer quickly so that it can be implemented quickly.
    B. Become the group leader and guide group members to complete the task using his solution.
    C. **Present his idea to the group and ask for alternative ideas.**
    D. Task group members with solving the problem consistent with his solution.

Performance Descriptor: Demonstrates responsibility for following safe practices, rules, procedures and etiquette in physical activity settings.

Sample Questions

7. When running a race with another person, it is safe practice to:
    A. Choose someone to race against who is slower than you.
    B. Run a longer race before a shorter race.
    C. **Give yourself slow-down space after the finish line.**
    D. Keep the lanes as close as possible.

8. The club head on your golf club is loose. What should you do?
    A. Make sure that you swing the club in a place where no one will be hurt if the club head comes off.
    B. Ask for some tape to fix it.
    C. Check to see whether it's loose enough to worry about.
    D. **Stop practice until you get a new club.**

9. Which of the following behaviors is **not** part of what it is to be a good sport?
    A. You play your best whether you are winning or losing.
    B. You let your opponents know when they have made a good play.
    C. You let everyone on your team have a chance to play.
    D. **You let the referee know when you have committed a foul even if it wasn't called.**

10. How should Samantha act when the official makes a call with which she disagrees?
    A. Let everyone know that it was a bad call.
    B. **Accept the official's call and play by the spirit of the game.**
    C. Point out the mistake to the official.
    D. Wait until after the game and then tell the official that it was a bad call.

11. What should you do if an opponent drops his/her racket accidentally during a competitive net game and he/she cannot play the point?
    A. Offer to replay the point.
    B. **Continue to play.**
    C. Stop play and give yourself a point.
    D. Declare that dropping a racket is a safety violation, which makes you the winner.

Performance Descriptor: Exhibits supportive behavior.

Sample Question

12. Good sportsmanship means that, when you win a game, you should:
    A. Not say or do anything.
    B. Thank the opposing team for a good game.
    C. Congratulate your teammates.
    D. Celebrate your win enthusiastically

Performance Descriptor: Recognizes the different benefits associated with participation in various types of physical activities.

Sample Questions

13. Of the following activities that Kaitlin enjoys regularly, which should she select if she wants the **most** fitness benefit?
    A. Lap swimming.
    B. Tai chi.
    C. Walking.
    D. Volleyball.

14. Charice wants to increase her participation in physical activity so that she is active every day. What criteria should she use for selecting an activity?
    A. Select the activity that her friends say they like to do.
    B. Select an activity that she doesn't know how to do.
    C. Select an activity that is enjoyable to her.
    D. Select the most popular activity among classmates.

15. Your Fitnessgram® test revealed that you need to improve your muscle strength. The **best** way for you to improve in this fitness component would be by:
    A. Jogging.
    B. Dance Dance Revolution.
    C. Weight training.
    D. Step aerobics.

16. Which would best serve to help Carla improve or maintain her flexibility?
    A. Weight training.
    B. Curl-ups.
    C. Line dancing.
    D. Gymnastics.

17. Devin's doctor has warned him of the risk factors associated with his obesity and has recommended that he improve his cardiorespiratory fitness. Devin should begin by:
    A. Taking a brisk evening walk every day.
    B. Jogging every day for 30 minutes.
    C. Completing 3 to 4 sprints down the football field 3 times a week.
    D. Jogging three times a week for 30 minutes.

18. If you really enjoy risk-taking activities, a good choice for participation would be:
    A. Bicycling.
    B. Kayaking.
    C. Karate.
    D. Soccer.

19. A major disadvantage of team sports for maintaining a physically active lifestyle is that they all:
    A. Require a lot of expensive equipment.
    B. Need to be performed indoors.
    C. Require other people to participate with you.
    D. Have to be played during the day.

20. Susan has moved to a new town and wants to become involved in a local softball league and ballroom dance class. Those activities promote primarily:
    A. Social interaction.
    B. Spending time alone.
    C. Risk-taking challenges.
    D. Competition.

21. Which one of the following lifestyle changes to improve physical activity doesn't require much effort and could improve your health?
    A. Taking the stairs instead of the elevator.
    B. Playing basketball at a local community league.
    C. Organizing a group to go on a backpacking trip.
    D. Working out to an exercise video every morning before going to school.

Performance Descriptor: Recognizes the attraction of participation in various physical activities.

Sample Questions

22. Tara's favorite physical activity is mountain biking. She might enjoy that activity most because:
    A. She enjoys a challenge and being outdoors.
    B. It requires inexpensive equipment.
    C. She can do it anywhere.
    D. She is not skilled at most other activities.

23. Your friend is not very active. How can you best encourage him to start exercising?
    A. Invite him to join you in an enjoyable activity.
    B. Show him a list of those activities that you believe are fun and challenging.
    C. Encourage him to seek the advice of athletes.
    D. Give him a handout from class on the benefits of being active.

24. Students who are physically active and watch what they eat usually:
    A. Earn better grades in school.
    B. Are not well liked by other students.
    C. Are healthier.
    D. Don't have a lot of free time.

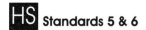

25. A good choice of physical activity for a person who wants to be physically active but hates sports that include running would be:
    A. Jogging.
    B. Dance.
    C. Soccer.
    D. Wii sports.

26. Other than health benefits, why would Carli value rock climbing, mountain biking and kayaking?
    A. Social interaction.
    B. The challenge.
    C. Self-expression.
    D. Cooperation.

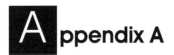

Appendix A

NASPE's National Standards for Physical Education And Secondary-Level Indicators & Assessment Tasks

Standard 1:
Demonstrates competency in motor skills and movement patterns needed to perform a variety of physical activities.

Middle School

Archery

Performance Indicator:

Perform the skills and tactics of individual competitive sports in a game-like situation.

Assessment Task:

Shoot arrows into the target from 10 yards.

Badminton

Performance Indicator:

Perform the skills and tactics of dual competitive sports in a game-like situation.

Assessment Task:

Play a competitive game of singles badminton.

Folk Dance

Performance Indicator:

Perform specific patterns and sequences in dance and rhythmic activities.

Assessment Task:

Perform a partner or group folk/ethnic/square dance.

Floor Hockey

Performance Indicator:

Perform the skills and tactics of team sports in a game-like situation.

Assessment Task:

Play a modified game of 3-v-2 floor hockey.

Line Dance

Performance Indicator:

Perform specific patterns and sequences in dance and rhythmic activities.

Assessment Task:

Perform a line dance.

Pickleball

Performance Indicator:

Perform the skills and tactics of dual competitive sports in a game-like situation.

Assessment Task:

Play a competitive game of singles pickleball.

Soccer

Performance Indicator:

Perform the skills and tactics of team sports in a game-like situation.

Assessment Task:

Play a modified game of 3-v-2 soccer.

Softball

Performance Indicator:

Perform the skills and tactics of team sports in a game-like situation.

Assessment Task:

Field a ground ball, throw a catchable ball and catch a catchable ball.

Team Handball

Performance Indicator:

Perform the skills and tactics of team sports in a game-like situation.

Assessment Task:

Play a modified game of 3-v-2 team handball.

Traverse Climbing

Performance Indicator:

Perform basic skills in adventure/outdoor activities.

Assessment Task:

Traverse a horizontal climbing wall.

Ultimate Frisbee®

Performance Indicator:

Perform the skills and tactics of team sports in a game-like situation.

Assessment Task:

Play a 3-on-3 modified game of Ultimate Frisbee®.

Volleyball

Performance Indicator:

Perform the skills and tactics of team sports in a game-like situation.

Assessment Task:

Overhead-pass and forearm-pass a tossed ball to a target player.

High School

Basketball

Performance Indicator:

Demonstrate competence in team court sports.

Assessment Task:

Play a 3-v-3 half-court basketball game.

Bowling

Performance Indicator:

Demonstrate competence in individual/dual competitive activities.

Assessment Task:

Bowl and score 10 frames, using an appropriate-weight ball.

Canoeing

Performance Indicator:

Demonstrate competency in adventure/outdoor activities.

Assessment Task:

Paddle a canoe through a 25-yard course.

Flag Football

Performance Indicator:

Demonstrate competence in team field sports.

Assessment Task:

Play a modified game of 3-v-3 flag football with a quarterback and two pass receivers on each team.

Golf

Performance Indicator:

Demonstrate competency in individual/dual competitive sports.

Assessment Task:

Demonstrate a pre-swing stance and a full swing in golf.

Soccer

Performance Indicator:

Demonstrate competence in team field sports.

Assessment Task:

Play a modified game of 3-v-3 soccer.

Swimming

Performance Indicator:

Demonstrate competency in individual/non-competitive sports.

Assessment Task:

Swim in both prone (face-down) and supine (face-up) positions and tread water.

Tennis

Performance Indicator:

Demonstrate competence in individual/dual sports.

Assessment Task:

Play 2 games or 6 minutes of tennis singles, whichever comes first.

Volleyball

Performance Indicator:

Demonstrate competency in team court sports.

Assessment Task:

Play a modified game of 4-v-4 volleyball.

Wall Climbing

Performance Indicator:

Demonstrate competence in adventure/outdoor activities.

Assessment Task:

Climb a vertical wall.

Weight Training

Performance Indicator:

Demonstrate competency in individual and non-competitive activities.

Assessment Task:

Perform and spot a bench press (free weight) exercise for 5-10 repetitions.

Standard 2:

Demonstrates understanding of movement concepts, principles, strategies and tactics as they apply to the learning and performance of physical activities.

Middle School

Performance Descriptor:

Explains critical elements of specialized skills.

Performance Descriptor:

Analyzes how positive transfer improves skill performance.

Performance Descriptor:

Examines how force and spin can alter the outcomes of skill performance.

Performance Descriptor:

Analyzes basic game strategies for invasion (e.g., ultimate, soccer), net (badminton, volleyball) and fielding (softball) games.

Performance Descriptor:

Analyzes the role of physical abilities in performance.

High School

Performance Descriptor:

Compares/contrasts critical elements of specialized skills originating from a common movement pattern.

Performance Descriptor:

Designs advanced game strategies for invasion, net, fielding and target activities.

Performance Descriptor:

Analyzes skill performance using biomechanical concepts.

Performance Descriptor:

Designs and justifies a practice plan using motor learning concepts.

Performance Descriptor:

Analyzes physical development across the lifespan that influences physical activity choices.

Standard 3:

Participates regularly in physical activity.

Standard 4:

Achieves and maintains a health-enhancing level of physical fitness.

Middle School

Performance Descriptor:

Participates in a variety of physical activities as part of a healthful lifestyle.

Performance Descriptor:

Demonstrates use of self-management skills related to maintaining a physically active lifestyle.

Performance Descriptor:

Participates in a variety of health-enhancing fitness activities to improve health-related physical fitness.

Performance Descriptor:

Evaluates current level of physical activity.

Performance Descriptor:

Achieves healthy levels of health-related, criterion-referenced standards for fitness.

Performance Descriptor:

Applies principles of training to improve and/or maintain the specific components of health-related fitness.

Performance Descriptor:

Assesses physiological indicators of exercise during and after physical activity.

Performance Descriptor:

Describes the relationship of cardiorespiratory fitness, muscle strength and endurance, and flexibility to body composition.

Performance Descriptor:

Applies principles of conditioning that enhance performance.

High School

Performance Descriptor:

Implements a personal physical activity plan that is part of a healthful lifestyle.

Performance Descriptor:

Employs self-management skills to maintain a physically active lifestyle.

Performance Descriptor:

Achieves levels of health-related criterion-referenced standards for fitness.

Performance Descriptor:

Demonstrates the skill, knowledge and desire to monitor and adjust activity levels to meet personal fitness needs.

Standard 5:

Exhibits responsible personal and social behavior that respects self and others in physical activity settings.

Standard 6:

Values physical activity for health, enjoyment, challenge, self-expression and/or social interactions.

Middle School

Performance Descriptor:

Applies procedures for keeping others and self safe during physical activity.

Performance Descriptor:

Describes problem-solving techniques to resolve conflicts.

Performance Descriptor:

Demonstrates concern for the rights and feelings of others in resolving conflicts.

Performance Descriptor:

Exhibits supportive verbal and nonverbal behavior toward peers of different gender, race, ethnicity and ability.

Performance Descriptor:

Values participating in physical activity because of the health benefits, personal enjoyment and/or social interaction.

Performance Descriptor:

Recognizes competition as a source of challenge.

Performance Descriptor:

Identifies personal preferences (e.g., enjoyment, fun, social interaction) as criteria for selecting physical activities.

High School

Performance Descriptor:

Describes appropriate leadership and followership behaviors.

Performance Descriptor:

Applies problem-solving techniques.

Performance Descriptor:

Demonstrates responsibility for following safe practices, rules, procedures and etiquette in physical activity settings.

Performance Descriptor:

Exhibits supportive behavior.

Performance Descriptor:

Recognizes the different benefits associated with participation in various types of physical activities.

Performance Descriptor:

Recognizes the attraction of participation in various physical activities.

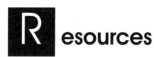

Resources

Published by the National Association for Sport and Physical Education:

Quality Physical Education Programs

- *Concepts and Principles of Physical Education: What Every Student Should Know* (2010)

- *Physical Activity and Sport for the Secondary School Student, 6th Edition* (2010)

- *Moving Into the Future: National Standards for Physical Education, 2nd Edition* (2004)

- *National Standards & Guidelines for Physical Education Teacher Education* (2009)

- *Quality Coaches, Quality Sports: National Standards for Athletic Coaches* (2006)

- *Physical Activity for Children: A Statement of Guidelines for Children Ages 5-12, 2nd Edition* (2003)

- *On Your Mark, Get Set, Go!: A Guide for Beginning Physical Education Teachers* (2004)

- *Coaching Issues & Dilemmas: Character Building Through Sport Participation* (2003)

- *Teaching Games for Understanding in Physical Education and Sport* (2003)

Opportunity to Learn Standards

- *Opportunity to Learn Guidelines for Elementary School Physical Education* (2009)

- *Opportunity to Learn Guidelines for Middle School Physical Education* (2009)

- *Opportunity to Learn Guidelines for High School Physical Education* (2009)

Appropriate Practices

- *Appropriate Practices in Movement Programs for Children Ages 3-5* (2009)

- *Appropriate Instructional Practice Guidelines for Elementary School Physical Education* (2009)

- *Appropriate Instructional Practice Guidelines for Middle School Physical Education* (2009)

- *Appropriate Instructional Practice Guidelines for High School Physical Education* (2009)

- *Appropriate Instructional Practice Guidelines for Higher Education Physical Activity Programs* (2009)

Assessment Series

- *Assessing and Improving Fitness in Elementary Physical Education* (2008)

- *Assessing Concepts: Secondary Biomechanics* (2004)

- *Assessing Student Outcomes in Sport Education* (2003)

- *Assessment in Outdoor Adventure Physical Education* (2003)

- *Assessing Heart Rate in Physical Education* (2002)

- *Authentic Assessment of Physical Activity for High School Students* (2002)

- *Elementary Heart Health: Lessons and Assessment* (2001)

- *Creating Rubrics for Physical Education* (2000)

- *Standards-Based Assessment of Student Learning: A comprehensive Approach* (1999)

Order online at www.naspeinfo.org or call (800) 321-0789

National Association for Sport and Physical Education

an association of the American Alliance for Health, Physical Education, Recreation and Dance

1900 Association Drive • Reston, Va. 20191

703-476-3410 • 703-476-8316 (fax) • www.naspeinfo.org

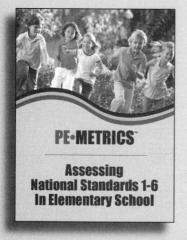
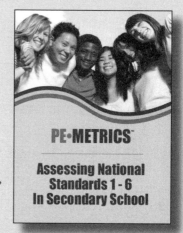

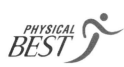
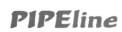
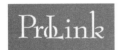
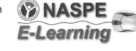

NASPE's Teacher Toolbox

Introduce your students to resources they will want to use after graduation.

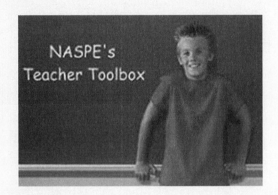

Students preparing for their student teaching experience will benefit from the FREE information available every month.

NASPE publishes a resource that features:

- FREE Downloads
- Lesson ideas that meet the national standards
- Physical activity break ideas
- Instant activities
- Parent letters promoting healthy lifestyle choices-in English and Spanish!
- Elementary and secondary fitness calendars for you to send home with your students-in English and Spanish!
- A special physical activity calendar for school staff or emerging exercisers
- Puzzles and games
- Coloring pages
- Employee wellness resources
- Family fun activities
- New NASPE resources and publications
- Information about the nation's health observances
- Latest resource materials for physical education and sports

Visit NASPE's Teacher Toolbox each month at www.naspeinfo.org
your one-stop shop for new teaching ideas!